How the IMMUNE SYSTEM *Works*

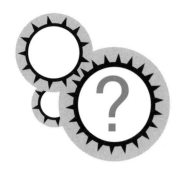

How the
IMMUNE SYSTEM
Works

LAUREN SOMPAYRAC, PhD

Retired Professor
Dept. of Molecular, Cellular, and Developmental Biology
University of Colorado
Boulder, Colorado

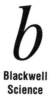

**Blackwell
Science**

©1999 by Blackwell Science, Inc.

Editorial Offices:
    Commerce Place, 350 Main Street, Malden, Massachusetts 02148, USA
    Osney Mead, Oxford OX2 0EL, England
    25 John Street, London WC1N 2BL, England
    23 Ainslie Place, Edinburgh EH3 6AJ, Scotland
    54 University Street, Carlton, Victoria 3053, Australia
Other Editorial Offices:
    Blackwell Wissenschafts-Verlag GmbH, Kurfürstendamm 57, 10707 Berlin, Germany
    Blackwell Science KK, MG Kodenmacho Building, 7-10 Kodenmacho Nihombashi, Chuo-ku, Tokyo 104, Japan

Distributors:

USA
    Blackwell Science, Inc.
    Commerce Place
    350 Main Street
    Malden, Massachusetts 02148
    (Telephone orders: 800-215-1000 or 781-388-8250; fax orders: 781-388-8270)
Canada
    Login Brothers Book Company
    324 Saulteaux Crescent
    Winnipeg, Manitoba, R3J 3T2
    (Telephone orders: 204-224-4068)
Australia
    Blackwell Science Pty, Ltd.
    54 University Street
    Carlton, Victoria 3053
    (Telephone orders: 03-9347-0300;
    fax orders: 03-9349-3016)
Outside North America and Australia
    Blackwell Science, Ltd.
    c/o Marston Book Services, Ltd.
    P.O. Box 269
    Abingdon
    Oxon OX14 4YN
    England
    (Telephone orders: 44-01235-465500;
    fax orders: 44-01235-465555)

Acquisitions: Chris Davis
Production and Typeset: Diane Lorenz, Lorenz Computer Graphics, Boulder, Co.
Manufacturing: Lisa Flanagan
Cover design by: Meral Dabcovich
Printed and bound by: Edwards Brothers, Ann Arbor, Mi.

Printed in the United States of America
99 00 01 02 5 4 3 2

First published 1999
ISBN: 0-632-04413-6

The Blackwell Science logo is a trade mark of Blackwell Science Ltd., registered at the United Kingdom Trade Marks Registry

The electron micrograph of the macrophage that appears on the cover and on page 6 was taken by Lennart Nilsson and obtained from Boehringer Ingelheim International GmbH.

The author would like to express his gratitude to Dr. Gilla Kaplan (Rockefeller University) for kindly providing the electron micrographs of the killer cell and its target that appear on page 11.

DEDICATION

I dedicate this book to my sweetheart, my best friend, and my wife: Vicki Sompayrac.

ACKNOWLEDGEMENT

I am indebted to Diane Lorenz for preparing all the figures in this book, for designing the logo, and for composing the text and figures in "camera ready" form. She has been a delight to work with.

I would like to thank the following people who have read various parts of this book and have offered their critical comments: Drs. Linda Clayton, Jim Cook, Tom Mitchell, Lanny Rosenwasser, and Dan Tenen. I would especially like to acknowledge the input of Dr. Mark Dubin, who read every page, and whose wise suggestions helped make this a much better book; and the work of Vicki Sompayrac, who helped purge the book of jargon, and whose editing was invaluable in preparing the final manuscript.

Finally, I would like to thank my editor at Blackwell, Chris Davis, who understood my dream to write an immunology book dedicated to students who were beginning to study the immune system. Instead of pressuring me to make the book more "mainstream," as most other editors would have done, Chris gently offered suggestions that helped make the dream a reality.

CONTENTS

HOW TO USE THIS BOOK

I wrote *How the Immune System Works* because I couldn't find a book that would give my students an overall view of the immune system. Sure, there are as many good, thick textbooks as a person might have money to buy, but these are crammed with every possible detail. There are also lots of "review books" that are great if you want a summary of what you've already learned -- but they won't teach you immunology. What was missing was a short book that tells, in simple language, how the immune system fits together -- a book that presents the big picture of the immune system without the jargon and the details.

How the Immune System Works is written in the form of "lectures," because I want to talk to you directly, just as if we were together in the classroom. This book is short, so you should be able to finish it in a few days. In fact, I strongly suggest that you sit down with this little book and read it from start to finish. The whole idea is to get an overall view of the subject, and if you read one lecture a week, that won't happen. Don't "study" the book the first time through -- just read it and enjoy. Later you can go back and re-read the appropriate lectures as your immunology course progresses -- to keep you from losing sight of the big picture as the details get filled in.

Although the first lecture is a light-hearted overview meant to give you a running start at the subject, you'll soon discover that this is not "baby immunology." *How the Immune System Works* is a concept-driven analysis of <u>how the immune system players work together</u> to protect us from disease -- and <u>why</u> they do it this way.

In some settings, *How the Immune System Works* will serve as the main text for the immunology section of a larger course. In a semester-long undergraduate or graduate immunology course, your professor may use this book either as a companion to a detailed text or as the central text, supplemented by additional readings.

No matter how your professor may choose to use this book, however, you should keep one important point in mind: I didn't write *How the Immune System Works* for your professor. This book's for <u>you</u>!

PART I

The Healthy Immune System

AN OVERVIEW

Immunology is a difficult subject to study for several reasons. First, there are lots of details, and sometimes these details get in the way of understanding the concepts. To get around this difficulty, we are going to concentrate on the big picture -- it will be easy for you to find the details somewhere else. A second difficulty in learning immunology is that there is an exception to every rule. Immunologists love these exceptions, because they give clues as to how the immune system functions. But for now, we're just going to learn the rules. Oh, sure, we'll come upon exceptions from time to time, but we won't dwell on them. Our goal will be to examine the immune system, stripped to its essence. The third difficulty in studying immunology is that our knowledge of the immune system is still evolving. As you'll see, there are many unanswered questions, and some of the things that seem true today will be proven false tomorrow. I'll try to give you a feeling for the way things stand now, and from time to time I'll discuss what immunologists speculate may be true; but keep in mind that, although I'll try to be straight with you, some of the things I'll tell you will change in the future (maybe even by the time you read this!).

Probably the main reason immunology is such a tough study, however, is that the immune system is really a "network" that involves many different players who interact with each other. Imagine you are watching a football game on TV, and the camera is isolated on one player, say, the tight end. You see this guy run full speed down the field, and then stop. It doesn't seem to make any sense. Later, however, you see the same play on the big screen, and now you understand. That tight end took two defenders with him down the field, leaving the running back uncovered to catch the pass and run for a touchdown. The immune system is just like that. It is a network of players who cooperate to get things done, and just looking at one player doesn't

make much sense -- you need an overall view. That's the purpose of this first lecture, which you might call "turbo immunology." Today, I'll take you on a brief tour of the immune system, so you can get a feeling for how it all fits together. Then in the next six lectures, we'll go back and take a more serious look at the players and their interactions.

PHYSICAL BARRIERS

Our first line of defense against invaders is a physical barrier. We tend to think of our skin as the main barrier, but in fact, the area covered by our skin is only about two square meters. In contrast, the area covered by the mucus membranes that line our digestive, respiratory, and reproductive tracts measures about 400 square meters. The point here is that there is a large perimeter that must be defended against attacks by viruses, bacteria, and parasites. To cause trouble, these invaders must first get past the physical barriers.

THE INNATE IMMUNE SYSTEM

Any invader that breaches the physical barrier of skin or mucosa is greeted by the innate immune system -- our second line of defense. Imagine you are getting out of your hot tub, and as you step onto the deck, you get a large splinter in your big toe. On that splinter are lots of bacteria, and within a few hours you'll notice (unless you had a lot to drink in that hot tub!) that the area around where the splinter entered is red and swollen -- indications that your innate immune system has kicked in.

In your tissues are roving bands of white blood

cells that defend you against attack. To us, tissue looks pretty solid -- that's because we're so big. To a cell, tissue looks more like a sponge with holes through which individual cells can move rather freely. One of the defender cells that is stationed in your tissues is the most famous innate immune system player of them all: the macrophage. If you are a bacterium, a macrophage is the last cell you want to see after your ride on that splinter. Here is an electron micrograph showing a macrophage about to devour a bacterium:

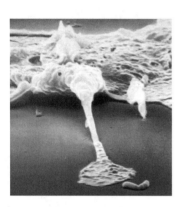

What you'll notice is that the macrophage is not waiting until it bumps into the bacterium. No, it's reaching out a foot to grab that bacterium, because bacteria and other invaders give off chemical signals that actually attract macrophages. When it encounters a bacterium, the macrophage first engulfs the bacterium in a pouch (vesicle) called a phagosome. This vesicle is then taken inside the cell where it fuses with another vesicle called a lysosome that contains powerful chemicals and enzymes which can destroy the bacterium. This whole process is called phagocytosis, and here is a series of "snapshots" that shows how it happens:

I should point out that macrophages are not very tidy eaters, and they frequently burp some of their meal back out into the tissues. This is important because this debris can signal other immune system players that the battle is on.

Why is this creature called a macrophage, you may be wondering. Well, "macro," of course, means large -- and the macrophage is a large cell. Phage comes from a Latin or Greek word (I can never remember which, and I suspect that you don't care) meaning "to eat." So a macrophage is a big eater. In fact, in addition to defending against invaders, the macrophage functions as a garbage collector. It will eat almost anything. Immunologists take advantage of this appetite by feeding macrophages iron filings. Then, using a small magnet, they can separate macrophages from other cells in a cell mixture. Really!

Where do macrophages come from? Macrophages and all the other blood cells are made in the bone marrow where they descend from self-renewing cells called stem cells -- the cells from which all the blood cells "stem." By self-renewing, I mean that when a stem cell goes through mitosis and divides into two daughter cells, it does a "one for me, one for you"-type thing in which some of the daughter cells go back to being stem cells, and some of the daughters go on to become macrophages or other kinds of blood cells. As each daughter cell matures, it has to make a lot of choices that determine which type of blood cell the daughter cell will be when it grows up. As you can imagine, these choices are not random, but are rather carefully controlled to make sure you have enough of each kind of blood cell. Here is a figure showing the many different kinds of blood cells (macrophage, neutrophil, eosinophil, etc.) a stem cell can become:

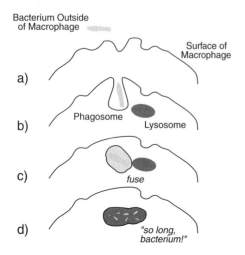

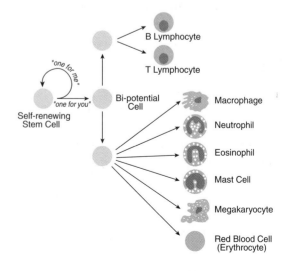

When macrophages first come out of the bone marrow and enter the blood stream, they are called monocytes. All in all you have about two billion of these "young macrophages" circulating through your blood at any one time, and you can be very glad they are there, because without them you'd be in deep trouble. Monocytes circulate in the blood for an average of about three days, during which time they are looking for a place to escape into the tissues. They travel to the capillaries, which represent the "end of the line" as far as blood vessels go, looking for a crack between the endothelial cells that line the capillaries. These cells look like shingles, and if the monocyte can get a foot between them, it can leave the blood, enter the tissues, and mature into a macrophage. In the tissues, most macrophages just hang out, do their garbage collecting thing, and wait for you to get that splinter, so they can do some real work.

When macrophages eat the bacteria on that splinter, they give off chemicals that constrict the blood vessels leading away from the point of entry, and the build-up of blood in this area is what makes your toe red. In addition, some of these chemicals cause the endothelial cells to contract, leaving spaces between them so that fluid in the capillaries can leak into the tissues. It is this fluid that causes the swelling. Also, during their battle with bacteria, macrophages produce proteins called cytokines. These function as hormone-like messengers which facilitate communication between cells of the immune system. Some of the cytokines alert other cells traveling in nearby capillaries that the battle is on, and influence these cells to exit the blood to help with the fight. Fragments of bacteria that macrophages have burped back into the tissues also serve as signals to recruit more defenders from the blood. Pretty soon you have a vigorous inflammatory response going on in your toe, as the innate immune system battles to eliminate the invaders.

When you think about it, this is a great strategy. You have a large perimeter to defend, so you station sentinels (macrophages) to patrol and check for invaders. These sentinels are armed and ready to fight. When a macrophage encounters an invader, it sends out signals that recruit more defenders to the site of the battle, and then it does its best to hold off the invasion until replacements arrive. Because the innate response involves players like macrophages that are "hard wired" to recognize a relatively small number of very common invaders, your innate immune system usually responds so quickly that the battle is over in just a few days.

There are other players on the innate team, and we will talk about them at length in the next lecture. For example, in addition to cells like the macrophage, which make it their business to eat invaders (the so-called "professional phagocytes"), the innate system includes the complement proteins that can punch holes in bacteria, and some rather mysterious cells called natural killer (NK) cells. These NK cells are able to kill bacteria, parasites, virus-infected cells, and cancer cells. The mystery is how they know what to kill.

THE ADAPTIVE IMMUNE SYSTEM

About 99% of animals get along just fine with only natural barriers and the innate immune system to defend them. However, for the fancy animals, the vertebrates, Mother Nature has laid on a third level of defense: the adaptive immune system. Opinions vary on why this extra level of protection is needed for vertebrates. Some say it's because these animals are more complex or because they have fewer offspring. There are even those who believe that the adaptive immune system was designed to protect us against cancer, but I'm not buying that. Cancer is mostly a disease of old age, and evolutionary pressure to survive decreases after animals have finished bearing and raising their young. No, it is most likely that the adaptive immune system evolved to protect us against viruses, because as you will see, the innate immune system isn't great against viruses.

As the name implies, the adaptive immune system can change to protect us against specific invaders. One of the first indications that such a system existed was back in the 1790's when Edward Jenner began vaccinating the English against smallpox virus. In those days, smallpox was a major health problem. Hundreds of thousands of people died from smallpox, and many more were horribly disfigured by the infection. What Jenner noticed was that milkmaids frequently contracted a disease called cowpox which caused lesions on their hands that looked similar to the sores caused by the smallpox virus. Moreover, Jenner noted that milkmaids who had had cowpox almost never got smallpox (which, it turns out, is caused by a close relative of the cowpox virus).

So Jenner decided to do a daring experiment. He collected pus from the sores of a milkmaid who had cowpox, and used this to inoculate a little boy named James Phipps. Later, when Phipps was re-inoculated with pus from the sores of a person infected with small-pox, he did not contract the disease. Incidentally, if you remember your Latin, you'll recall that the word for cow is vacca -- which explains where we got the word vaccine. History makes out the hero in this affair to be Edward Jenner, but you and I know that the real hero that day was the young boy. Imagine having this big man approach you with a large needle and a tube full of pus! Although this isn't the kind of experiment you could do today, we can be thankful that Jenner's exper-iment was a success, because it paved the way for vac-cinations that have saved countless lives.

One important point about this smallpox vacci-nation is that it only protected against smallpox. Phipps was still able to get mumps, measles, and the rest. As you will see, this is one of the hallmarks of the adaptive immune system: it adapts to defend against specific invaders.

ANTIBODIES AND B CELLS

Eventually, immunologists determined that immunity to smallpox was due to some small proteins that circulated in the blood of immunized individuals. These proteins were named antibodies, and the agent that elicited the antibodies was called the antigen -- in this case, the cowpox virus. Here's a sketch that shows what the prototype antibody, immunoglobulin G (IgG), looks like:

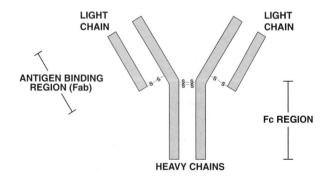

As you can see, each antibody molecule is made up of two pairs of two different proteins, heavy chain and light chain. What is interesting about antibodies is that they are divalent and bifunctional. By divalent, I mean that each IgG antibody is able to grab (bind to) two antigens at the same time -- that is, it has two "hands." The antibody is bifunctional, because in addition to binding antigen with its hands, the Fc portion of the antibody (the legs, if you will) can bind to special recep-tors (Fc receptors) on the surfaces of cells like macrophages. Although IgG makes up about 75% of the antibodies in the blood, there are four other classes (isotypes) of antibodies: IgA, IgD, IgE, and IgM. The function of a given class of antibody depends on its Fc region, because that part of the molecule determines which cell types the antibody will bind to. All anti-bodies are made by B cells: white blood cells that are born in the bone marrow, and then mature into anti-body factories called "plasma" B cells.

For a given antibody molecule, the two antigen binding regions will bind to the same antigen (i.e., the "hands" are identical), so to bind to many different antigens, many different antibody molecules are required. Now, if we expect antibodies to protect us from every possible invader (and we do), how many different antibodies would we need? Well, immunolo-gists have made rough estimates that about 100 million should do the trick. Since each antigen binding region is composed of a heavy chain and a light chain, we could mix and match about 10,000 different heavy chains and 10,000 different light chains to get the 100 million different antibodies we need. But how can B cells generate 100 million different antibody molecules without using every gene in the B cell? You see, current estimates of the total number of genes in a human cell range from about 20,000 to 100,000, so if each heavy and light chain were encoded by a different gene, you would quickly use up a lot (perhaps all!) of the genes in the cell. You see the problem.

Two main theories were put forth to explain how B cells could make such a diverse collection of antibodies. The first held that B cells display on their surfaces a generic antibody molecule that would fold itself around the antigen. Then -- and this was the magic part -- the B cell would somehow be instructed to make lots more antibodies that looked just like the fold-ed one on its surface. This idea sounds pretty goofy today, but back then immunologists were frantic to find some way of explaining antibody diversity.

CLONAL SELECTION

The other theory was called clonal selection. We now call it the clonal selection "principle," because we believe it is correct. Clonal selection holds that each B cell makes antibodies that have only one type of antigen binding (Fab) region, and therefore are specific for a certain antigen, called its "cognate" antigen. These antibodies are displayed on the surface of the B cell, and it is through these surface antibodies (called B cell receptors) that the B cell is able to know that its cognate antigen is "out there." You see, cells are basically blind to what is going on outside them, so they use antenna-like receptors that span the cell membrane to recognize certain molecules on the outside, and to relay this information to the inside of the cell. In this way cells are able to sense the environment in which they live and react to it.

There are lots of different receptors on every cell, and they are "tuned" to recognize and bind to different molecules. The B cell receptor (BCR) is tuned to recognize and bind to its cognate antigen, and when this recognition takes place, the B cell proliferates to make a lot more identical B cells that can make antibodies which recognize that same antigen. It takes about twelve hours for a B cell to double in size and divide into two daughter cells, and this period of proliferation usually lasts about a week. At the end of this time, there will be roughly 20,000 B cells, all of which have antibodies on their surfaces that can recognize the same antigen. Most members of this clone will then mature into plasma B cells which will produce and export (secrete) huge quantities of antibodies into the blood and tissues. Thus, when a B cell recognizes its cognate antigen, that B cell is selected to proliferate in order to make a clone of B cells, all with the same specificity. This clonal selection principle is recognized as one of the major concepts in immunology.

ANTIBODY DIVERSITY

Okay, so each B cell makes only one kind of antibody, but we are still stuck with the problem of how to make 100 million different B cells that can be selected, when needed, to protect us against all possible invaders. This riddle was finally solved in 1977 by Susumu Tonegawa, who received the Nobel Prize for his discovery. When Tonegawa started working on this

problem, the dogma was that the DNA in every cell in the body was the same. This made perfect sense, because after the egg is fertilized, the DNA in the egg is copied, and these copies are passed down to the daughter cells, where they are copied again, and passed down to their daughters, etc. Therefore, barring errors in copying, each of our cells should end up with the same DNA as that fertilized egg. Tonegawa, however, hypothesized that although this is probably true in general, there might be exceptions. His idea was that all of our B cells might start out the same, but as they mature, changes in the antibody genes might take place, and these changes might be enough to generate the 100 million different antibodies we need. He decided to test this hypothesis by comparing the DNA sequence of the light chain from a mature B cell with the DNA sequence of the light chain from an immature B cell. Sure enough, he found they were different, and they were different in a very interesting way. What Tonegawa and others discovered was that the mature immunoglobulin genes are made by modular design. For example, the DNA for the heavy chain in the immature B cell includes four types of modules (V, D, J, and C), and there are multiple copies of these modules (gene segments), each of which is slightly different. In the human, there are about 100 different V segments, at least four different D segments, six different J segments, etc. To make a mature heavy chain, the B cell chooses (more or less at random) one of each kind of segment and pastes them together like this:

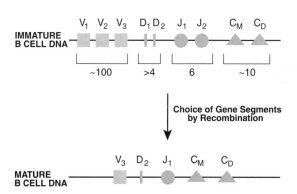

You have seen this kind of mix and match strategy used before to create diversity. For example, to create the many different proteins, twenty different amino acids are mixed and matched. To create genetic diversity, chromosomes you inherited from your mother and father are mixed and matched to make your egg or sperm cells. Once Mother Nature gets a good idea, she uses it over and over -- and this modular design idea is one of her best!

It turns out that there are enough modules to mix and match to create about 10 million different combinations of heavy and light chains -- not quite enough. So, to make things even more diverse, when the gene segments are joined together, additional DNA bases are added or deleted. When this junctional diversity is included, there is no problem in creating 100 million B cells, each of which can make a different antibody. The magic of this scheme is that by using modular design and junctional diversity, only a small number of gene segments (about 300) is required to create incredible antibody diversity.

ANTIBODIES -- HOW THEY FUNCTION

Now that you know how antibodies are made, we need to talk about what they do. Interestingly, although antibodies are very important in the defense against invaders, they really don't kill anything. Their job is to plant the "kiss of death" on an invader -- to tag it for destruction. If you go to a fancy wedding, you will usually pass through a receiving line before you are allowed to have at the champagne. Of course, one of the functions of this receiving line is to introduce everyone to the bride and groom. But the other function is to be sure no outsiders are admitted to the celebration. As you pass through the line, you will be screened by someone who is familiar with all of the invited guests. If she finds that you do not belong there, she will call the bouncer to have you removed. She doesn't do it herself -- certainly not. Her role is to identify undesirables, not to show them the door. It's the same with antibodies: They identify invaders, and let other players do the dirty work.

In developed countries, the most bothersome invaders are bacteria and viruses, and antibodies can bind to both to tag them for destruction. Immunologists like to say that antibodies can "opsonize" these invaders. This term comes from a German word that means "to prepare for eating." I like to equate opsonize with "decorate," because I imagine these bacteria and viruses with antibodies hanging all over them, decorating their surfaces. Anyway, when antibodies opsonize bacteria and viruses, they do so with their Fab regions, leaving their Fc regions available to bind to Fc receptors

on the surface of cells like macrophages. This way, antibodies can form a bridge between the phagocyte (e.g., a macrophage) and the invader, bringing the invader in close, and preparing it for eating (phagocytosis). This drawing depicts what I mean:

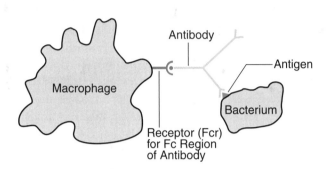

In fact, it is even better than this, because binding of the opsonized invaders to the Fc receptors of phagocytes increases their appetite, making them even more phagocytic. For viruses, antibodies can do another neat thing. Viruses are intracellular parasites that enter our cells by binding to certain receptor molecules on the cell surface. Of course, these receptors are not placed there for the convenience of the virus. They are normal receptors, like the Fc receptor, that have quite legitimate functions, but which the virus has learned to use to its own advantage. Once inside the cell, the virus uses the cellular machinery to make many copies of itself. These newly-made viruses then burst out of the cell, sometimes killing it, and go on to infect neighboring cells. Now the neat part. Frequently, antibodies are made that bind to the part of the virus that plugs into the cellular receptor. These are called "neutralizing" antibodies. Once a neutralizing antibody binds to a virus, that virus is no longer able to "dock" on the surface of the cell. As a result, the virus is left outside the cell, opsonized and ready to be eaten by phagocytes.

T CELLS

Now, you may have realized that there is a flaw in the antibody defense against viruses: Once the virus gets into the cell, the antibody can't get to it, so the virus is safe to make thousands of copies of itself. Mother Nature also recognized this problem, and to deal with it, she invented the famous "killer T cell," another member of the adaptive immune system team.

The importance of T cells is suggested by the fact that in a human, there are about a trillion of them. T cells are very similar to B cells in appearance. In fact, even under a microscope, an immunologist can't tell them apart. Like B cells, T cells are produced in the bone marrow, and they display on their surfaces an antibody-like molecule called the T cell receptor (TCR). Like the B cell's receptor (the antibody molecule attached to its surface), the TCR is also made by a mix and match, modular strategy. As a result, TCRs are about as diverse as BCRs. T cells also obey the principle of clonal selection: Each T cell makes only one kind of TCR, and when that TCR binds to its cognate antigen, the T cell proliferates to build up a clone of T cells with the same specificity. This proliferation takes a week or more to complete, so like the antibody response, the T cell response is slow and specific.

There are important differences between B and T cells, however. Whereas the B cell matures in the bone marrow, the T cell matures in the thymus (that's why it is called a "T" cell). Further, although B cells make antibodies that can recognize any organic molecule, T cells recognize only protein antigens. In addition, the B cell can secrete its receptors in the form of antibodies, whereas the TCR stays tightly glued to the surface of the T cell. Perhaps most importantly, a B cell can recognize an antigen "by itself," whereas a T cell, like an old English gentleman, will only recognize an antigen if it is "properly" presented by another cell. I'll tell you what this means in a bit.

There are at least two, and probably three kinds of T cells: helper T cells, killer T cells (usually called cytotoxic lymphocytes -- CTLs for short), and suppressor T cells. Immunologists are not too sure about these suppressor T cells, and there is still some question as to whether they actually exist as a separate T cell type. Although it is clear that something must turn the immune system off after invaders have been repulsed, the question of whether or not a special T cell does this is being hotly debated.

The killer T cell is a weapon that most immunologists feel has evolved to deal with virus-infected cells. The most dramatic way it does this is by using a protein called perforin to perforate virus-infected cells -- literally to bore holes in them. The net result is that the virus-infected cell is killed, and the virus within the cell dies with it. In these micrographs, you can see the hole a CTL has made in its target cell:

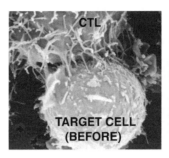
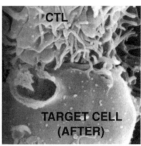

The other kind of "for real" T cell is the helper T cell (Th). As you will see, this cell serves as the quarterback of the immune system team -- it directs the action by secreting protein molecules called cytokines that have dramatic effects on other immune system cells. These cytokines have names like interleukin 2 (IL-2) and interferon gamma (IFN-γ), and we will discuss what they do in later lectures. For now, it is only important to realize that plasma B cells are antibody factories and helper T cells are cytokine factories.

ACTIVATION OF THE ADAPTIVE IMMUNE SYSTEM

Because B and T cells are such potent weapons, Mother Nature put into place the requirement that cells of the adaptive immune system must be activated before they can function. Collectively, B and T cells are called lymphocytes, and how they are activated is one of the key issues in immunology. We'll talk about activation in some detail in Lectures Three and Five, but for now I want to sketch how helper T cells are activated, because many features of this activation are typical of how other lymphocytes are activated.

The first step in the activation of a helper T cell is recognition of its cognate antigen. Remember that T cell receptors only recognize antigen that is properly presented by another cell, and it turns out that only certain cells can do this presentation. These special cells are called antigen presenting cells (APCs for short). Macrophages, for example, are excellent antigen presenting cells, but only a macrophage that has "eaten" the Th cell's cognate antigen will be able to activate the helper T cell. So the first signal that a Th cell needs for activation is very specific: recognition of its cognate antigen presented by an antigen presenting cell. This drawing shows a Th cell contacting a macrophage that is presenting its cognate antigen:

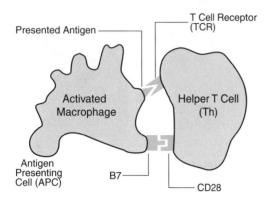

Specific recognition of presented antigen, however, is not sufficient to activate a Th cell -- a second signal or "key" is also required. This signal is non-specific (it's the same for any antigen), and involves a protein on the surface of the APC (B7 in this drawing) that plugs into its receptor on the surface of the Th cell (CD28 in the drawing). You see an example of this kind of two-key system when you visit your safe deposit box. You bring with you a key that is specific for your box -- it won't fit any other. The bank teller provides a second, master key that will fit all the boxes. Only when both keys are inserted into the locks on your box can it be opened. Your specific key alone won't do it, and the teller's non-specific key alone won't either. You need both. Now, why do you suppose Th and other cells of the adaptive immune system require two keys for activation? For safety, of course -- just like your bank box. These cells are powerful weapons that must only be activated at the appropriate time.

Once a helper T cell is activated, it proliferates to build up a clone of Th cells with the same TCR specificity, and these Th cells then mature into cells that can produce cytokines. This should start to sound pretty familiar by now: activation, proliferation, and maturation.

A COMPARISON OF THE INNATE AND ADAPTIVE IMMUNE SYSTEMS

At this point, I want to pause to emphasize the difference between the innate and adaptive immune systems. Imagine that you are in the middle of town and someone steals your shoes. Maybe you are wearing those fancy running shoes that every mugger wants.

Anyway, you look around for a store where you can buy another pair, and the first store you see is called Charlie's Custom Shoes. This store has shoes of every style, color, and size, and the salesperson is able to fit you in exactly the shoe you need. However, when it comes time to pay, you are told that you will have to wait a week or two to get your shoes -- they will have to be custom-made for you, and that will take a while. But you need shoes now, you complain. You are barefoot, and you at least need something to put on your feet until those custom shoes arrive! So they send you across the street to Freddie's Fast Fit -- a store that has only a few styles and sizes. Freddie's wouldn't be able to fit Michael Jordan, but Freddie's does have shoes in the common sizes that fit most people, so you can get a pair to tide you over.

This is just the way the adaptive and innate immune systems work. The adaptive system has B cells that can make antibodies to fit every possible antigen, but antibodies have to be custom-made according to the principle of clonal selection. As a result, you have to wait a week or two for these antibodies. In the meantime, you need something to fight off that invader or at least hold it at bay until the antibodies arrive. This is where the innate system comes in. Its players (like the macrophage) are already in place, and they are ready to defend against the common invaders you are likely to meet on a day-to-day basis. In fact, in many instances, the innate system is so effective and so fast that the adaptive immune system never even kicks in.

Until recently, immunologists thought that the only real function of the innate system was to provide a rapid defense that would hold off invaders until the adaptive immune system could get cranking. However, it is now clear that the innate system does much more than that. The innate system has evolved receptors that detect the presence of the common pathogens we encounter in daily life -- viruses, bacteria, fungi, and parasites. In contrast to the innate system, whose receptors are precisely tuned to detect common invaders, the adaptive immune system's receptors are totally unfocused -- they are so diverse that they can probably recognize any organic molecule in the universe. As a result of this receptor diversity, the adaptive system is clueless as to which molecules are dangerous and which are not. So how does the adaptive system distinguish friend from foe? The answer is that it relies on the innate system. In a real sense, the innate system gives "permission" to the adaptive system to respond to an invasion. In fact, it's even better than that. Not only does the innate system alert the adaptive system to danger, the innate system also instructs the adaptive system on which weapons to use and exactly where in the body these weapons should be deployed! I'll tell you more about this exciting new development in Lecture Five.

ANTIGEN PRESENTATION

One thing we need to clear up is exactly how antigen is presented to T cells. It turns out that for presentation, the protein antigen is first chewed up into small pieces called peptides, and these peptides are then presented in the grasp of molecules called major histocompatibility complex proteins (MHC for short). As you know, "histo" means tissue, and these MHC molecules, in addition to being presentation molecules, are also responsible for rejection of transplanted organs. When you hear that someone is waiting for a "matched" kidney, this is what the transplant surgeon is trying to match: MHC molecules.

There are two types of MHC molecules that are commonly used for presentation of peptides, and these are called class I and class II. Class I molecules are found in varying amounts on most cells in the body. Whereas class I MHC molecules are rather ubiquitous, class II MHC molecules are usually found only on specialized cells that can present antigen (e.g., macrophages). Here is an artist's conception of what these MHC molecules look like:

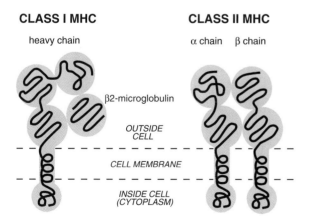

Although MHC I is made up of one long chain (the heavy chain) plus a short chain (β2-microglobulin), and MHC II has two long chains (α and β), you'll notice right away that these molecules look very similar. Because it's hard to visualize the real shapes of these molecules from drawings like this, I've made a few pictures that I think will help. Here is an image of what an empty MHC molecule might look like from the viewpoint of the T cell receptor:

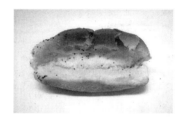

You can see right away where the fragment of the protein would fit into the groove. Next, we see what a fully-loaded, class I molecule might look like:

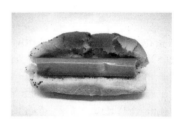

I can tell it's class I because the peptide fits nicely into the groove. It turns out that the ends of the class I molecule are closed, so the peptide must be about nine amino acids in length to fit in properly. Class II molecules are slightly different:

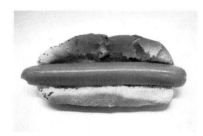

Here you see that the peptide overflows the groove. This works fine for class II, because the ends of the groove are open, so protein fragments as large as about fifteen amino acids fit nicely.

I always think of MHC molecules as "billboards." MHC I displays what is going on <u>inside</u> the cell. For example, inside a virus-infected cell, viral proteins are chopped up into small peptides, loaded onto MHC I molecules, and transported to the surface, where they are displayed for killer T cells (CTLs) to look at. This is the way CTLs get to look "into" a cell to check whether it is infected and should be destroyed.

MHC II molecules also function as billboards, but in this case they display what is going on <u>outside</u> the antigen presenting cell. For example, during a bacterial infection, macrophages eat some of the bacteria, cut the bacterial proteins up into small pieces, load these peptides onto class II molecules, and display them on the surface for helper T cells to see. Because many invaders never enter a cell (e.g., most bacteria), this system with two types of billboards works great, because it lets T cells have a look at both intracellular and extracellular invaders -- so all the bases are covered.

THE SECONDARY LYMPHOID ORGANS

If you've been thinking about how the adaptive immune system might get turned on during an attack, you've probably begun to wonder whether this could ever happen at all. There are probably only about 10,000 T cells that will have TCRs specific for a given invader, and for these T cells to be activated, they must come in contact with an antigen presenting cell that has also "seen" the invader. Given that these T cells and APCs are spread all over the body, it would seem very <u>un</u>likely that this would happen before the invasion was completely out of hand. It's all just too improbable.

Fortunately, to make this system work with reasonable probability, Mother Nature invented the "secondary lymphoid organs," the most well known of which is the lymph node. You may not be familiar with the lymphatic system, so I'd better say a few words about it. In your home, you have two plumbing systems. The first involves the water that comes out of your faucet. This is a pressurized system with the pressure being provided by a pump. In addition, you also have another plumbing system that includes the drains in your sinks, showers, and toilets. This system is not under pressure -- the water in this system just flows down the drain and out into the sewer. The two systems are connected in the sense that eventually, the

waste water is recycled and used again.

The plumbing in a human is very much like this. We have a pressurized system in which blood is pumped around the body by the heart. Everybody knows about this one. But we also have another plumbing system, the lymphatic system. This system is not under pressure, and it drains the fluid (called lymph) that leaks out of our blood vessels into our tissues. Without this system, our tissues would fill up with fluid and we'd look very puffy. Fortunately, lymph is collected from our tissues, and is transported by muscular contraction through a series of one-way valves to the upper torso, where it is recycled back into the blood. From this diagram, you can see that as the lymph winds its way back to empty into the blood, it passes through a series of way stations, the lymph nodes:

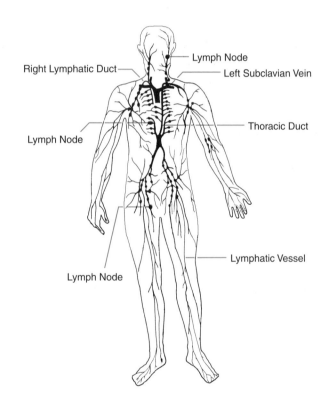

There are thousands of lymph nodes that range in size from very small to almost as big as a Brussels sprout. These lymph nodes function as "dating bars" -- places where T cells, B cells, and APCs gather to communicate and to be activated. In addition, because foreign antigens like bacteria and viruses can be carried by the lymph to nearby nodes, this system allows T and B cells to sample foreign antigens that are present "in the neighborhood." By bringing together T cells, B cells, APCs, and antigen in the small volume of a lymph node, Mother Nature increases the probability that they will interact to activate the adaptive immune system. In Lecture Six, we'll talk more about lymph nodes and the other secondary lymphoid organs.

IMMUNOLOGICAL MEMORY

After B and T cells have been activated, have proliferated to build up clones with identical antigen specificities, and have vanquished the enemy, most of them die off. This is a good idea, because we wouldn't want our immune systems to fill up with old B and T cells. On the other hand, it would be nice if some of these experienced B and T cells would stick around, just in case we were exposed to the same invaders again. That way, the adaptive immune system wouldn't have to start from scratch. And that's just the way it works. These "leftover" B and T cells are called memory cells, and in addition to being more numerous than the original, inexperienced B and T cells, these memory cells are also easier to activate. As a result of this immunological memory, the adaptive system usually can spring into action so quickly that you never even experience any symptoms during a second attack. Although it is clear that many of the vaccinations we receive as children generate memory cells that protect us throughout our lives, immunologists are still debating exactly how this immunological memory is maintained. In Lecture Three we'll discuss the current thinking on this issue.

TOLERANCE TO SELF

As we discussed earlier, B cell receptors and T cell receptors are so diverse that they can recognize any potential invader. This raises a problem, however, because if the receptors are this diverse, many of them are certain to recognize our own "self" molecules (e.g., the proteins that make up our cells or proteins that circulate in our blood). If this were to happen, our adaptive immune system might attack our own bodies, and we could die from autoimmune disease. Fortunately, Mother Nature has devised ways to educate B cells and T cells to discriminate between self and non-self.

Exactly how lymphocytes are taught to be tolerant of self is still being studied intensively, and when this important riddle is finally solved, a Nobel Prize will certainly be awarded. What is known so far is that there are several different ways of teaching B and T cells not to attack our own molecules. As a result, serious attacks on self that would result in autoimmune disease are quite rare.

EPILOGUE

We have come to the end of our turbo overview of the immune system, and by now you should have a rough idea of who the players are and how the system works. In the next six lectures, we will focus more sharply on the individual players of the innate and adaptive systems, paying special attention to how and where these players interact with each other to make the system function efficiently. Then, in the final lectures, we will examine the role of the immune system in disease.

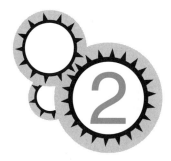

2 THE INNATE IMMUNE SYSTEM

Until recently, most immunologists didn't pay much attention to the innate system, perhaps because the adaptive system seemed more exciting. However, studies of the adaptive immune system have led to a new appreciation of the role that the innate system plays, not only as a second line of defense (if we count physical barriers as our first defense), but also as an activator and a controller of the adaptive response.

The importance of the innate system's quick response to common invaders is easy to understand if you think about what could happen in an uncontrolled bacterial infection. Imagine that the splinter from your hot tub deck introduced just one bacterium into your tissues. As you know, bacteria can multiply very quickly. In fact, a single bacterium doubling in number every thirty minutes could give rise to roughly 100 trillion bacteria in one day. If you've ever worked with bacterial cultures, you know that a one liter culture containing one trillion bacteria is so dense that you can't see through it. So, a single bacterium proliferating for one day could yield a dense culture of about 100 liters. Now realize that your total blood volume is only about five liters, and you can appreciate what an unchecked bacterial infection could do to a human!

The innate immune system includes the complement proteins, professional phagocytes, and natural killer cells. We'll begin our discussion with one of my favorites:

THE COMPLEMENT SYSTEM

The complement system is composed of about twenty different proteins that work together to destroy invaders and to signal other immune system players that the attack is on. When I first read about the complement system, I thought it was way too complicated to even bother understanding, but as I studied it further, I began to realize that it is really quite simple and beautiful. Complement proteins start to be made during the first trimester of fetal development, so it's clear that Mother Nature wants this important system to be ready to go, well before a child is born. Indeed, those rare humans born with a defect in one of the complement proteins do not live long before succumbing to infection.

As with just about everything else in the immune system, the complement system must be activated before it can function, and there are three ways this can happen. The first, the so-called "classical" pathway, depends on antibodies for activation, so we'll leave this for a later lecture. The complement system does the same thing, independent of how it is activated, so you won't miss much by having to wait until later to hear about the antibody-dependent pathway of activation. The second way the complement system can be activated is called the "alternative" pathway, although in evolutionary terms, this pathway certainly evolved before the classical pathway. Immunologists call the antibody-dependent system classical, simply because it was discovered first. Until recently, immunologists thought that these were the only two ways the complement system could be activated. However, a third mode of activation has now been discovered: the "lectin" activation pathway.

THE ALTERNATIVE PATHWAY

The proteins that make up the complement system are produced mainly by the liver, and are very abundant in blood and tissues. The most abundant complement protein is called C3. In the chemical environment of the blood and tissues, C3 molecules are continuously being clipped (cut) to yield two smaller proteins. One of the protein fragments created by this "spontaneous" reaction, C3b, is very reactive, and can bind to two common chemical groups (amino or hydroxyl groups). Because many of the proteins and carbohydrates that make up the cell surfaces of invaders have amino or hydroxyl groups, there are lots of targets for these little C3b "grenades."

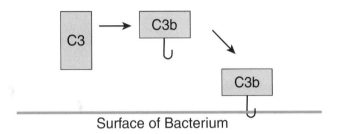

If C3b doesn't react with one of these groups within about sixty microseconds, it is neutralized by binding to a water molecule, and the game is over. So the spontaneously-clipped C3 molecule has to be right up close to the surface of a cell in order for the complement cascade to continue. Once C3b is stabilized by binding to the cell surface, another complement protein, B, binds to C3b, and complement protein D comes along and clips off part of B to yield C3bBb.

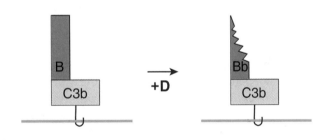

Now the fun begins. Imagine a bacterium that has had one of these grenades explode nearby, and now has this C3bBb molecule glued to its surface. It turns out that C3bBb acts like a "chain saw" that can cut C3 proteins and convert them to C3b. As a result, other C3 molecules don't have to wait for another spontaneous clipping event to be converted to C3b -- the C3bBb molecule (called a convertase) can do the job very efficiently. Once another C3 molecule has been clipped, it too can bind to an amino or hydroxyl group on the bacterial surface.

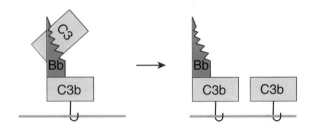

This process can continue, and pretty soon there will be lots of C3b molecules attached to the surface of the target bacterium -- and each of them can form the C3bBb convertase which can then cut even more C3 molecules. As you can see, a positive feedback loop has been set up here, and now the whole thing just snowballs:

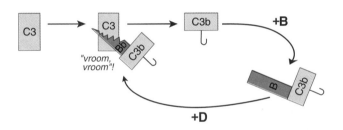

Once C3b is bound to the surface of a bacterium, the complement cascade can proceed further. The C3bBb chain saw can cut off part of another complement protein, C5, and the clipped product, C5b, can combine with other complement proteins (C6, C7, C8, and C9) to make a "membrane attack complex" (MAC for short). To do this, C5b, C6, C7, and C8 form a "stalk" that will anchor the complex in the bacterial cell wall, and C9 proteins are then added to make a channel that opens up a hole in the surface of the bacterium.

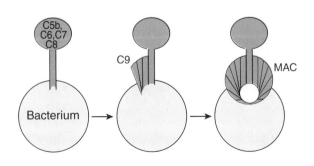

Do you remember the picture from last lecture of the hole that a killer T cell (CTL) had created in its target cell? Well, the perforin protein produced by the CTL is a close relative of the C9 complement protein. Like a virus-infected cell that has been attacked by perforin, once a bacterium has holes in its surface, the game is over.

Now, you are probably wondering: With all these grenades going off all over the place, why doesn't the complement system form MACs on the surface of our own cells? The answer is that a number of safeguards keep this from happening. First, there is a protein on the surface of human cells called decay accelerating factor (DAF) which accelerates the breakdown of the convertase, C3bBb, by other proteins in the blood. This can keep the positive feedback loop from getting started, since C3bBb is the convertase that converts C3 to C3b. Moreover, C3b can be clipped to an inactive form by proteins in the blood, and this clipping is accelerated by an enzyme that is present on the surface of human cells. There is yet another protein, CD59 (also called protectin), on human cells that can kick almost-finished MACs off the cell surface before they can poke a hole. Obviously, Mother Nature was so worried about the complement system reacting inappropriately that she evolved multiple mechanisms to control it.

There's an interesting example that illustrates why these controls are so important. As you know, transplant surgeons don't have enough human organs to satisfy the demand for transplantation, so they are considering using organs from other animals. One of the hot candidates for organ donors is the pig, because pigs are cheap to raise, and their organs are about the same size as those of humans. As a warm-up for human transplantation, the surgeons decided to transplant a pig organ into another primate, a baboon. The result was not a big success. Almost immediately, the baboon's immune system began to attack the organ, and within minutes the transplanted organ was a bloody pulp. The culprit? The complement system. It turns out that the pig versions of DAF and CD59 don't work to control primate complement, so the unprotected pig organ was vulnerable to attack by the baboon complement system.

This story highlights two important features of the complement system. First, the complement system works very fast. These complement proteins are present at high concentrations in blood and in tissues, and they are ready to go against any invader that has a surface with a spare hydroxyl or amino group. A second characteristic of this system is that if a cell surface is not protected, it will be attacked by complement. In fact, the picture you should have is that the complement system is continually dropping these little grenades, and any surface that is not protected against complement attack will be a target. In this system, the default option is death.

THE LECTIN ACTIVATION PATHWAY

In addition to the classical and alternative pathways of complement activation, there is a third, recently-discovered pathway that may be the most important activation pathway of all. The central player in this pathway is a protein that is produced mainly in the liver, and which is present in moderate concentrations in the blood and tissues. This protein is called mannose-binding lectin (MBL for short). A lectin is a protein that is able to bind to a carbohydrate molecule, and mannose is a carbohydrate molecule found on the surface of many common, disease-causing agents (pathogens). For example, mannose binding lectin has been shown to bind to yeasts such as *Candida albicans*, to viruses such as HIV and influenza A, to many bacteria including *Salmonella* and *Streptococci*, and to parasites like *Leishmania*. In contrast, mannose-binding lectin does not bind to the carbohydrates found on healthy human cells and tissues.

The way mannose-binding lectin works to activate the complement system is very simple. In the blood, MBL complexes with (binds to) another protein called MASP. When the mannose-binding lectin binds to its target (mannose on the surface of a bacterium, for example), the MASP protein functions like a convertase to clip C3 complement proteins to make C3b. Because C3 is so abundant in the blood, this happens very efficiently. The C3b fragments can then bind to the surface of the bacterium, and the complement chain reaction we just discussed is off and running.

Whereas the alternative activation pathway is spontaneous, and can be visualized as "grenades" randomly going off here and there, the lectin activation pathway can be thought of as "smart bombs" that are directed to their targets by the mannose-binding lectin. The targeting of MASP to a carbohydrate on the surface of an invader is an example of an important strategy employed by the innate system: The innate system mainly focuses on carbohydrate molecules that make up the cell walls of common pathogens.

OTHER FUNCTIONS OF THE COMPLEMENT SYSTEM

In addition to building membrane attack complexes, the complement system has two other functions in innate immunity. When C3b has attached itself to the surface of an invader, it can be clipped by a serum protein to produce a smaller fragment, iC3b. The "i" prefix denotes that this cleaved protein is now inactive for making MACs. However, it is still glued to the invader, and it can prepare the invader for phagocytosis (can opsonize it) in much the same way that invaders can be opsonized by antibodies. On the surface of phagocytes (e.g., macrophages) are complement receptors that can bind to iC3b, and the binding of iC3b-opsonized invaders makes macrophages even more phagocytic. Thus, a second function of complement is to act like a poor man's antibody in opsonization.

The complement system has a third important function. Fragments of complement proteins can serve as chemoattractants -- chemicals that recruit other immune system players to the site of the battle. For example, C3a and C5a are the pieces of C3 and C5 that are clipped off when C3b and C5b are made (let nothing be wasted!). Both C3a and C5a are active in attracting macrophages and neutrophils. Interestingly, these fragments are called anaphylatoxins, because they can contribute to anaphylactic shock -- something we will talk about in another lecture.

So you see, the complement system is quite versatile. It can destroy invaders by building MACs. It can enhance the function of phagocytic cells by tickling their complement receptors. And it can signal other cells that the attack is on. Most importantly, it can do all these things very fast.

THE PROFESSIONAL PHAGOCYTES

The second arm of the innate system is composed of the professional phagocytes. Last lecture, I talked briefly about one of these, the macrophage. Now let's take a closer look at this, the most versatile of the professional phagocytes.

THE MACROPHAGE

Macrophages can exist in three stages of readiness. In tissues, macrophages are usually found just lounging and slowly proliferating. In this "resting" state, they function primarily as garbage collectors, taking sips of whatever is around them, and keeping our tissues free of debris. While resting, they express very few class II MHC molecules on their surfaces, so they aren't much good at presenting antigen to T cells. This makes sense. Why would they want to present garbage anyway? For the average macrophage, life is pretty boring. They live for months in tissues and just collect garbage.

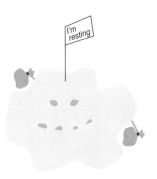

Every once in a while, however, some of these resting macrophages receive signals which alert them that the barrier defense has been penetrated, and that there are intruders in the area. When this happens, they become activated (or "primed," as immunologists usually say). In this state, macrophages begin to take larger gulps, and they upregulate expression of class II MHC molecules. Now, if they do happen to engulf invaders, the macrophages can function as antigen presenting cells, and can display fragments of the invader's proteins (peptides) on their surfaces.

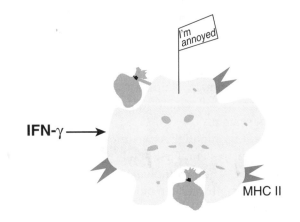

Although it is likely that a number of different signals can prime a resting macrophage, the best studied signal is an intercellular communication molecule (a "cytokine") called interferon gamma (IFN-γ). You may know that there are three kinds of interferons: α, β, and γ. The α and β interferons are proteins that are made and exported (secreted) by cells in response to a viral infection. One function of IFN-α and IFN-β is to warn nearby cells that they may soon be attacked by viruses, and that if they are, they must commit suicide. As a result of this altruistic act, the infected cells and the viruses within them die together. Most cells can make IFN-α and IFN-β, so this is a very important defense against viruses. In contrast, IFN-γ, sometimes called immune interferon, is a signaling molecule that is primarily secreted by T cells and NK cells.

In the primed state, macrophages are good antigen presenters and reasonably good killers. However, they have an even higher state of readiness, "hyperactivation," that they can attain if they receive a direct signal from an invader. The best studied signal is conveyed by a molecule called lipopolysaccharide (LPS for short). LPS is found in the outer cell wall of Gram-negative bacteria like *E. coli*. LPS is shed by bacteria, and can bind to receptors on the surface of primed macrophages. Macrophages also have receptors for mannose -- the carbohydrate that is an ingredient of the cell walls of many common pathogens and which, as we discussed earlier, is a "danger signal" that can activate the complement system. When receptors on the surface of the macrophage bind to either LPS or mannose, the macrophage knows for sure that there has been an invasion. Faced with this realization, the macrophage stops proliferating, and focuses its attention on killing.

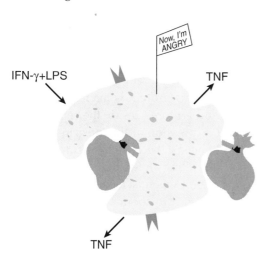

In the hyperactive state, macrophages grow larger and increase their rate of phagocytosis. In fact, they become so large and phagocytic that they can ingest invaders that are as big as unicellular parasites. When hyperactivated, macrophages produce and secrete the cytokine, TNF. This cytokine can kill tumor cells and virus-infected cells, and can also help activate other immune system cells. Inside the hyperactivated macrophage, the number of lysosomes increases, so that killing of ingested invaders becomes more efficient. In addition, hyperactivated macrophages increase production of reactive oxygen molecules like hydrogen peroxide. You know what peroxide can do to hair, so you can imagine what it might do to a bacterium! Finally, when hyperactivated, a macrophage can kill multicellular parasites that are even larger than it is by partially ingesting them and then dumping the contents of its lysosomes onto the parasite. A hyperactivated macrophage is a killing machine!

So macrophages are very versatile cells. They can function as garbage collectors, as antigen presenting cells, and as vicious killers. However, you should not get the impression that macrophages have three "gears." Nothing in immunology has gears, and the activation state of the macrophage is a continuum that really depends on both the type and the strength of the activation signals it receives.

THE NEUTROPHIL

Although the macrophage is unmatched in versatility, the most important of the professional phagocytes is probably the neutrophil. Neutrophils make up about 70% of the white blood cells in circulation, and about 100 billion of these cells are produced each day in our bone marrow. Clearly they must be important or we wouldn't have so many of them. Neutrophils live a very short time. They come out of the bone marrow programmed to die in an average of about five days. Interestingly, they die by committing suicide, a process known as "apoptosis." In contrast to macrophages, neutrophils are not antigen presenting cells -- they are professional killers that exit blood vessels and enter the tissues, ready to kill.

My friend, Dan Tenen, studies neutrophils. His wife, Linda Clayton, who studies T cells, likes to kid him by asking, "Why do you study neutrophils? All they do is dive into pus and die!" She's right, of course

-- pus is mainly dead neutrophils. However, Dan reminds her that humans can live for long periods without those fancy T cells, but without neutrophils, they will succumb to infection and die within a matter of days.

As neutrophils exit the blood, they become activated, and in this state, they are very similar to hyperactivated macrophages. They are incredibly phagocytic, and once their prey has been taken inside, a whole battery of powerful chemicals awaits the unlucky "guest." Now, I want to ask you a question: Why do you think Mother Nature set things up so that macrophages are very long lived, yet neutrophils live only a few days? Doesn't that seem wasteful? Why not let these neutrophils enjoy a long life, just like the macrophages? That's right! It would be too dangerous! Neutrophils come out of the blood vessels ready to kill, and in the course of this killing, there is always damage to normal tissues. To limit the damage, neutrophils are programmed to be short lived. If the battle requires more neutrophils, more can be recruited from the blood -- there are plenty of them there. In contrast, you want macrophages to live a long time, because they act as sentinels that watch for invaders and signal the attack. When the battle is over, and macrophages stop receiving activation signals, those that have not died from exertion can actually revert back to the resting state, and resume collecting garbage.

You may be wondering, if neutrophils are all that dangerous, how do they know when to leave the blood and where to go? It certainly wouldn't do to have neutrophils leave the blood and become activated just any old place. No indeed, and the way this works is really neat. In the blood, neutrophils exist in an inactive state, and they are swept along by the blood at a high rate of speed: about 1000 microns per second. If you are the size of a neutrophil, that's really fast.

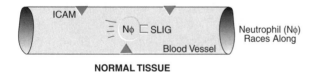

NORMAL TISSUE

In this sketch, you will notice there is a protein, ICAM (short for intercellular adhesion molecule), that is expressed on the surface of the endothelial cells that line blood vessels. There is also another adhesion molecule called selectin ligand (SLIG) that is expressed on the surface of neutrophils. As you can see, however, these two adhesion molecules are not "partners," so they don't bind to each other, and the neutrophil is free to zip along with the flowing blood.

Now imagine that you get a splinter in your big toe, and the bacteria on the splinter activate macrophages that are standing guard in the tissues of your foot. These activated macrophages give off "alarm" cytokines, interleukin 1 (IL-1) and TNF, that are designed to signal that an invasion has begun. When endothelial cells that line nearby blood vessels receive these alarm signals, they begin to express a new protein on their surfaces called selectin (SEL). It normally takes about six hours for this protein to be made and transported to the surface of endothelial cells. Selectin is the adhesion partner for selectin ligand, so once selectin is expressed on the endothelial cell surface, it functions like Velcro to grab neutrophils as they fly by. However, this interaction between selectin and its ligand is only strong enough to cause neutrophils to slow down and roll along the inner surface of the blood vessel.

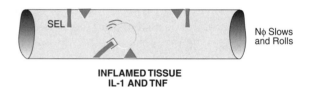

INFLAMED TISSUE
IL-1 AND TNF

As the neutrophil rolls, it "sniffs." What it's sniffing for is a signal that there is a battle (an inflammatory reaction) going on in the tissues. The complement fragment, C5a, and the bacterial wall component, LPS, are two of the inflammatory signals that the neutrophil recognizes. When it receives these signals, the neutrophil rushes a new protein called integrin (INT) to its surface. Lots of this protein is made in advance by the neutrophil, and is stored inside the cell until needed. To be useful, expression of the integrin proteins on the surface has to be fast, because the neutrophil hasn't stopped -- it's still rolling along. If it rolls too far, it will get outside the region where selectin is expressed, and the neutrophil will start to zoom along again at "blood speed." Once on the neutrophil's surface, integrin can interact with its binding partner, ICAM, which is expressed on the surface of endothelial cells. This interaction is very strong, and it causes the neutrophil to stop rolling.

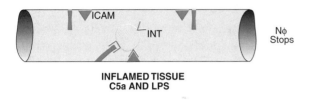

INFLAMED TISSUE
C5a AND LPS

Once the neutrophil has stopped, it can be influenced by molecules called chemoattractants to pry apart the endothelial cells that line the blood vessels, exit into the tissues, and migrate to the site of inflammation. These chemoattractants include our old friend from the complement system, C5a, as well as fragments of bacterial proteins called f-met peptides.

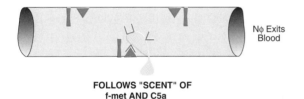

FOLLOWS "SCENT" OF
f-met AND C5a

All bacterial proteins begin with a special initiator amino acid called formyl methionine, (f-met) which less than .01% of human proteins contain, so f-met peptides are relatively unique to bacteria. As they ingest bacteria, macrophages burp up f-met peptides, so neutrophils that have exited the blood can follow the trail of f-met peptides to find the battle. In addition, cytokines such as TNF activate neutrophils as they travel through the tissues, so they arrive at the battle scene ready to kill.

You remember I mentioned that to completely upregulate expression of that first cellular adhesion molecule, selectin, takes about six hours. Why do you think it takes so long? That's right. Before you start to recruit reinforcements from the blood, you want to be sure that the attack is serious. If a macrophage encounters only a few invaders, it can usually handle the situation without help in a short time. In contrast, a major invasion involving many macrophages can go on for

days. The sustained expression of alarm cytokines from many macrophages engaged in battle is required to upregulate selectin expression, and this insures that more troops will be summoned only when they are really needed.

The second feature of this system that I'd like you to notice is that although neutrophils represent about 70% of the cells in the blood, there are very few neutrophils outside the blood vessels in normal tissues (i.e., tissues that are not infected). These cells are "on call." And who does the calling? The sentinel cell, the macrophage, of course. So you have this great system where a garbage collector alerts the "hired guns" when their help is needed. It is this cooperation between the macrophage and the neutrophil that makes the whole thing work.

This system -- which involves selectin-selectin ligand binding to make the neutrophil roll, integrin-ICAM interactions to stop the neutrophil, and chemoattractants and their receptors on the neutrophil to facilitate exit from the blood -- may seem a little over-complicated. Wouldn't it be simpler just to have one pair of adhesion molecules (say, selectin and its ligand) do all three things? Yes, it would be simpler, but it would also be very dangerous. In a human there are about 100 billion endothelial cells. Suppose one of them gets a little crazy, and begins to express a lot of selectin on its surface. If selectin binding were the only requirement, neutrophils could empty out of the blood into normal tissues where they could do terrible damage. Having three types of molecules that must be expressed before neutrophils exit the blood helps make the system fail safe.

Neutrophils are not the only blood cells that need to exit the blood and enter tissues. For example, eosinophils and mast cells, which are involved in protection against parasites, must exit the blood at sites of parasitic infection. Monocytes, which will eventually become tissue macrophages, also need to leave the blood stream at appropriate places. T cells and B cells must exit the blood and enter lymph nodes where they can be activated, and once activated, these lymphocytes must exit the blood into tissues at sites of infection. This whole business is like a mail system in which there are lots of packages (immune system cells) that must be delivered to the correct destinations.

Now here is the neat part. It turns out that all immune system cells use the same strategy as neutrophils to exit the blood. However, the Velcro-like molecules that cause the cells to roll and stop are different from cell type to cell type and destination to destination. As a result, these adhesion molecules actually can serve as "zip codes" to insure that cells are delivered to the appropriate locations. You see, the selectins and their ligands are really families of molecules, and only certain members of the selectin family will pair up with certain members of the selectin ligand family. The same is true of the integrins and their ligands. Because of this two-digit zip code (type of selectin, type of integrin), there are enough "addresses" available to send the many different immune system cells to many different destinations. By equipping immune system cells with different adhesion molecules and by equipping their intended destinations with the corresponding adhesion partners, Mother Nature can insure that immune system cells will roll, stop, and exit the blood exactly where they are needed.

NATURAL KILLER CELLS

In addition to the complement system and the professional phagocytes, there is a third important player on the innate immune system team -- the natural killer (NK) cell. This has been a difficult cell for immunologists to study, because there are different kinds of NK cells with somewhat different properties. These cells were originally called large granular lymphocytes, because, like the professional phagocytes, they are full of granules that contain chemicals and enzymes. Although NK cells are descended from stem cells just like the rest of the blood cells, it is still uncertain just where NK cells fit on the family tree. The most recent evidence suggests that they are in the same family as the lymphocytes (T and B cells), but they also have some similarities to macrophages.

Like neutrophils, NK cells use the "roll, stop, exit" strategy to leave the blood and enter tissues at sites of infection. Once in the tissues, NK cells are quite versatile. They can kill tumor cells, virus-infected cells, bacteria, parasites, and fungi -- and they have at least two methods of killing. First, they can bore a hole in a target cell by secreting perforin molecules to form a membrane attack complex on the surface of the target. NK cells can then secrete enzymes that enter the target cell and cause it to commit suicide. As their second weapon of destruction, NK cells can use a protein called Fas ligand (FasL) that is expressed on the NK cell

surface. FasL can interact with a protein called Fas on the surface of the target, and when these two proteins connect, they can signal the target cell to commit suicide by apoptosis.

One of the mysteries about NK cells is how they identify which cells to kill. Their method of target recognition is quite different from that of T cells, which recognize their targets through their T cell receptors. NK cells have no TCRs, so they must be looking at something besides peptides displayed by MHC proteins. The latest thinking is that killing by NK cells actually requires two signals -- a "kill" signal and the absence of a "don't kill" signal.

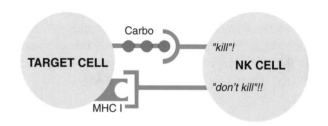

The "don't kill" signal seems to be the expression of MHC I molecules on the surface of the potential target, because cells that express MHC I usually can't be killed by NK cells. The "kill" signal is thought to involve interactions between proteins on the surface of the NK cell and special carbohydrates on the surface of the target. Presumably, the carbohydrate molecules act as flags that indicate the cell has been infected with a virus or has become a tumor cell, but this part is still poorly understood. The best current synthesis of this two-signal system is that the balance between the "kill" and the "don't kill" signals determines whether NK cells will kill a target cell.

Now, why do you think it would be a good idea to have NK cells kill targets that do not express MHC molecules? Well, you remember from the introductory lecture that killer T cells (CTLs) recognize foreign peptides presented by MHC proteins. So suppose some clever virus or cancer cell decides to turn off expression of these MHC molecules. Then that virus-infected cell or cancer cell would be invisible to the CTL, right? Well, it turns out that this is exactly what many viruses and cancer cells do -- downregulate MHC expression. So, in those cases, wouldn't it be great to have another weapon that would kill virus-infected or cancer cells that <u>don't</u> have MHC on their surfaces? You bet it would. And that's something NK cells do: they specialize in killing cells that lack MHC molecules on their surfaces.

NK cells have a couple of other interesting features. First, in contrast to T cells, which need to be educated not to attack self, NK cells are genius cells that don't need this education. Somehow, probably through recognition of the "kill" carbohydrate, the NK cell knows an invader when it sees one. It is also interesting that NK cells are rather like CTLs and helper T cells all rolled into one. NK cells use perforin and FasL to kill, just like CTLs, but in addition, NK cells can function as cytokine factories, much like Th cells. Indeed, NK cells are one of the major suppliers of IFN-γ.

In some ways, NK cells also resemble macrophages. They contain lots of lysosome-like granules, and they can exist in several stages of readiness. Resting NK cells are able to produce some IFN-γ and can kill, but they produce more IFN-γ and kill a lot better if they are activated. So, what activates these killers? Several signals have been identified that can activate NK cells. One is the bacterial cell wall component, LPS, that we learned earlier could activate macrophages. In addition, NK cells can be activated by the alarm interferons, IFN-α and IFN-β, that cells give off when they are under viral attack. Certainly, other signals will be discovered that can activate NK cells, but you get the idea: NK cells are activated by signals that indicate an attack is on.

THE INNATE IMMUNE SYSTEM -- A COOPERATIVE EFFORT

To make the innate system work efficiently, there must be cooperation between players on the innate system team. For example, there are two cytokines that help determine how much IFN-γ NK cells give off: TNF and interleukin 12 (IL-12). Whereas signals like LPS tell the NK cell to shift to a higher state of activation, TNF and IL-12 actually act like accelerators -- the more TNF and IL-12 NK cells receive, the more IFN-γ they make. And where do the accelerating factors, TNF and IL-12, come from? Why, from activated macrophages. So the IFN-γ needed to prime macrophages comes from NK cells, and the TNF and IL-12 required to increase the amount of IFN-γ made by

NK cells come from macrophages. As a result of this interdependence, macrophages and NK cells work together to get each other fired up. Here's how it works:

During a bacterial infection, molecules like LPS bind to receptors on the NK cell surface, and this signals that an attack is on. NK cells respond by producing significant amounts of IFN-γ.

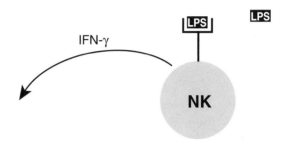

The IFN-γ produced by NK cells can prime macrophages, which can then be hyperactivated when their receptors also bind to LPS.

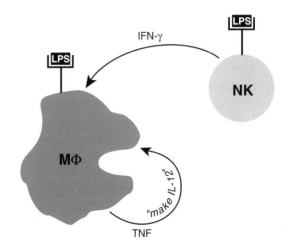

When a macrophage is hyperactivated, it produces lots of TNF. The macrophage also has receptors on its surface to which this cytokine can bind. When the TNF produced by the hyperactivated macrophage binds to these receptors, the macrophage begins to secrete another cytokine, IL-12. Together, TNF and IL-12 cause NK cells to produce even more IFN-γ, so that even more macrophages can be primed.

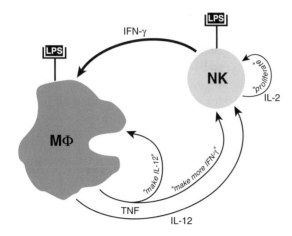

Now, there is something else neat going on here. IL-2 is a growth factor that is produced by NK cells, and which can cause these cells to proliferate. Normally, however, NK cells don't express the receptor for IL-2, so they are unable to respond to this cytokine, even though they are making it. Fortunately, macrophages can fix this problem, because TNF from the macrophage upregulates expression of IL-2 receptors on the surface of NK cells. Consequently, NK cells can now respond to the IL-2 they make and begin to proliferate, and as a result of this proliferation, there will soon be many more NK cells to defend against the invader.

So here you have these two cells, the macrophage and the NK cell, cooperating to set up a positive feedback loop. This positive feedback loop produces a "snowball" effect that helps the innate system respond quickly and strongly to destroy invaders.

This interaction between macrophages and NK cells is an excellent example of cooperation between the innate system players. Another example is the cooperation between the complement system and the professional phagocytes. As you learned earlier, complement protein fragments such as C3b can opsonize invaders for phagocyte ingestion. But complement opsonization can also play a role in activating macrophages, because when C3b binds to its receptor on the surface of a macrophage, it can provide an activation signal similar to that provided by LPS. This is a good idea, because there are invaders that can be opsonized by complement, but which do not make LPS.

Cooperation between the complement system and the phagocytes is not a one-way street. Activated macrophages actually produce several of the most

important complement components: C3, factor B, and factor D. This can be a big advantage, because in the heat of battle, complement proteins may be depleted, and macrophages can help resupply the complement system. In addition, in an inflammatory reaction, macrophages secrete chemicals that can increase the permeability of nearby blood vessels. As a result, these vessels become leaky. And what do you think leaks out into the tissues? More complement proteins!

Although in this lecture we have focused on cooperation between players on the innate immune system team, in subsequent lectures you will see that there is a great deal of cooperation between the innate system and the adaptive system. In fact, in most cases, the adaptive system will not respond to an invader unless the innate system has already recognized that there is danger.

HOW THE INNATE SYSTEM DEALS WITH VIRUSES

When viruses enter (infect) human cells, they take over the cell's machinery and use it to produce many more copies of the virus. Eventually, these newly-made viruses burst out of the infected cells, and go on to infect other cells in the neighborhood. We have already discussed some of the weapons the innate system can use to defend against viruses that are outside of cells. For example, the proteins of the complement system can opsonize viruses for phagocytosis by macrophages and neutrophils. In addition, for enveloped viruses like HIV, complement proteins can poke holes in the virus by constructing membrane attack complexes on the surface of the virus.

Although the innate system is quite effective against viruses outside the cell, the weapons the innate immune system can bring to bear on virus-infected cells are rather limited. This is a major problem, because each virus-infected cell can produce thousands of new viruses. NK cells and activated macrophages secrete cytokines like IFN-γ and TNF that in some cases can reduce the amount of virus that infected cells produce. Secreted TNF can kill some virus-infected cells, and cells infected by certain viruses can be killed by NK cells and activated macrophages.

All in all, complement, professional phagocytes, and NK cells do an okay job of dealing with a viral infection, especially in the early stages. However, viruses replicate quickly in virus-infected cells, and viruses are very clever -- many have discovered ways of evading the innate immune system. It is probably for this reason that Mother Nature invented the adaptive immune system -- the subject of our next three lectures.

SUMMARY FIGURE

In this figure, I have summarized some of the concepts we discussed in this lecture. For clarity, I have chosen a macrophage as a representative of the professional phagocytes, a bacterium as an example of an invader that exists outside human cells, and a virus as an example of a parasite that must enter a human cell to complete its life cycle. After each of the next three lectures, I will expand this figure to include the players from the adaptive immune system as they take the field.

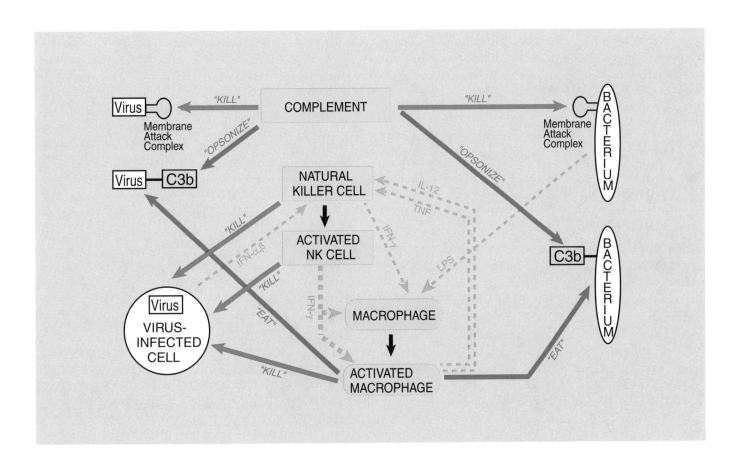

3   B CELLS AND ANTIBODIES

REVIEW

Let's quickly review the material we covered in the last lecture. We talked about the complement system of proteins, and how complement fragments can function as "poor man's antibodies" to tag invaders for ingestion by professional phagocytes. In addition, complement fragments can act as chemoattractants to help recruit phagocytic cells to the site of the battle. Finally, the complement proteins can participate in the construction of membrane attack complexes that can puncture and destroy certain bacteria and viruses.

The complement proteins are present in high concentrations in the blood and also in the tissues, so they are always ready to go. In addition, activation by the alternative (spontaneous) pathway simply requires that the complement protein fragment, C3b, bind to an amino or hydroxyl group on an invader. Because these chemical groups are ubiquitous, the default option in this system is death -- any surface that is not protected against binding by complement fragments will be targeted for destruction.

In addition to the alternative activation pathway, which can be visualized as "grenades" going off randomly here and there, there is a second pathway for activating the complement system that is more directed: the lectin activation pathway. In this system, a protein called mannose-binding lectin binds to carbohydrate molecules that make up the cell walls of common pathogens. Once bound, the mannose-binding lectin sets off the complement chain reaction on the surface of the invader. So the mannose-binding lectin can be thought of as a "smart bomb" that directs the complement system to invaders that have distinctive carbohydrate molecules on their surfaces.

We also talked in the last lecture about two professional phagocytes: macrophages and neutrophils. In the tissues, macrophages have a relatively long lifetime. This makes sense, because macrophages act as sentinels that patrol the periphery, checking for invaders. If they find an invader, they can be activated to become vicious killers. In their activated state, macrophages also can present antigen to T cells. After the battle has been won, macrophages that have not died can "de-activate" and go back to patrolling the perimeter.

Whereas macrophages are quite versatile, neutrophils really do only one thing -- kill. Neutrophils use cellular adhesion molecules to exit blood vessels at sites of inflammation, and as they exit, they are activated to become killers. Fortunately, these killers only live about five days. This limits the damage they can do to healthy tissues once an invader has been vanquished. On the other hand, if the attack is prolonged, there are plenty more neutrophils that can exit the blood and help out, since neutrophils represent about 70% of the circulating white blood cells.

Another player on the innate system team is the natural killer cell. These cells are a cross between a killer T cell and a helper T cell. Like CTLs, they can kill virus-infected cells by perforating the surface of the cell, or by triggering the apoptotic death program. Like helper T cells, NK cells can secrete cytokines that affect the function of both the innate and the adaptive immune systems.

In summary, the innate immune system provides a fast and effective response to common invaders. For the most part, players on the innate system team are "hard wired" to react to carbohydrate molecules that are unique to disease-causing agents (pathogens) or pathogen-infected cells. Phagocytes, NK cells, and complement proteins can attack immediately, because these weapons are already in place. As the battle continues, cooperation between players increases to strengthen the defense, and signals given off by the innate system recruit even more defenders from the blood stream.

The innate system also plays a crucial role in alerting the adaptive immune system to danger, so as we start to examine the adaptive system, you should be on the lookout for interactions between the two systems. I think you'll soon appreciate that the innate system does much more than just react quickly to common invaders.

B CELLS

We will begin our discussion of the adaptive immune system by focusing on one of its most important players: the B cell. Like all the other blood cells, B cells are born in the bone marrow, where they are descended from stem cells. About one billion B cells are produced each day during the entire life of a human, so even old guys like me have lots of freshly-made B cells. During their early days in the marrow, B cells select gene segments coding for the B cell receptor (BCR). These segments are assembled to make a complete gene, and the BCR encoded by this gene is then displayed on the surface of the cell where it can receive signals. The antibody molecule is almost identical to the B cell receptor, except that it lacks the protein sequences that anchor the BCR to the outside of the cell. Lacking this anchor, the antibody molecule is exported out of the B cell (is secreted), and therefore is free to travel around the body to do its thing. I want to tell you a little about the process of selecting gene segments to make a B cell receptor, because I think you'll find it interesting -- especially if you like to gamble.

THE B CELL RECEPTOR

The BCR is made up of two kinds of proteins, the heavy chain (Hc) and the light chain (Lc), and each of these proteins is encoded by genes that are assembled from gene segments. The gene segments that will be chosen to make up the final Hc gene are located on chromosome fourteen, and each B cell has two chromosome fourteens (one from Mom and one from Dad). This raises a bit of a problem, because as we discussed earlier, each B cell makes only one kind of antibody. Therefore, because there are two sets of Hc segments, it will be necessary to "silence" the segments on one chromosome fourteen to keep from getting two different Hc

proteins made by the same B cell. Of course, Mother Nature could have chosen to make one chromosome a "dummy," so that the other would always be the one that was used to make the Hc protein -- but she didn't. That would have been too boring. Instead, she came up with a much sweeter scheme, which I picture as a game of cards with the two chromosomes as players. It's a game of "winner takes all," in which each chromosome tries to rearrange its cards (gene segments) until it finds an arrangement that works. The first player to do this wins.

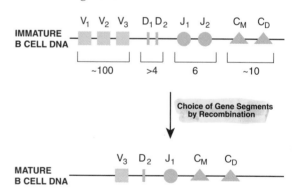

You remember from the first lecture that the finished heavy chain protein is made from four gene segments (V, D, J, and C), and that lined up along chromosome fourteen are multiple, slightly-different copies of each kind of segment.

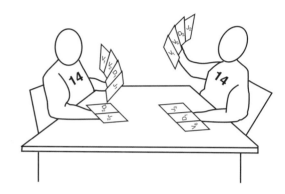

The players in this card game first choose one each of the possible D and J segments, and these are joined together by deleting the DNA sequences in between them. Then one of the many V segments is chosen, and this "card" is joined to the DJ segment, again by deleting the DNA in between. Next to the rearranged J segment is a string of gene segments that code for various constant regions. By default, the constant regions for IgM and IgD are used to make the BCR, just because they are first in line. Immunologists call these joined-together gene segment a "gene rearrangement," but it is really more the result of cutting and pasting than rearranging. Anyway, the chosen V, D, and J segments and the constant region segments all end up adjacent to each other on the chromosome.

Next, the rearranged gene segments are tested. What's the test? As you know, protein translation stops when the ribosome encounters one of the three stop codons, so if the gene segments are not joined up just right ("in frame"), the protein translation machinery will encounter a stop codon and terminate protein assembly right in the middle of the Hc. If this were to happen, the result would be a useless little piece of protein. In fact, you can calculate that each player has only about one chance in nine of assembling a winning combination of gene segments that will produce a full-length Hc protein. Immunologists call such a combination of gene segments a "productive rearrangement." If one of the chromosomes that is playing this game ends up with a productive rearrangement, the winning Hc protein is made and transported to the cell surface where it signals to the losing chromosome that the game is over. Exactly how the signal is sent and how it stops the rearrangement of gene segments on the other chromosome remain to be discovered.

Since each player has only about a one in nine chance of success, you may be wondering what happens if both chromosomes fail to assemble gene segments that result in a productive rearrangement. Well, the B cell dies. That's right, it commits suicide! It's a high stakes game, because a B cell that cannot express a receptor is totally useless.

If the heavy chain rearrangement is productive, the light chain players step up to the table. The rules of this game are very similar to the rules of the heavy chain game except that there is a second test which must be passed to win: the completed heavy and light chain proteins must fit together properly to make a complete antibody. If the B cell fails to productively rearrange heavy and light chains, or if the two chains don't match up correctly, the B cell commits suicide. So every mature B cell produces one and only one kind of BCR or antibody, made up of one and only one kind of Hc and Lc. Because of the mix and match strategy that is used to make the final Hc and Lc genes, the receptors on different B cells are so diverse that collectively, they can probably recognize any organic molecule that could exist. When you consider how many molecules

that might be, the fact that a simple scheme like this can create such diversity is truly breathtaking.

HOW THE BCR SIGNALS

The region of an antigen that the BCR recognizes is called the "epitope." For example, if the antigen is a protein, the epitope is the tiny region of that protein (usually six to twelve amino acids) that the BCR actually binds to. The function of the BCR is to recognize the epitope for which it is matched, and to signal this recognition to the nucleus of the B cell, so that genes involved in activation can be turned on or off. But how does this BCR "antenna" send a signal to the nucleus that it has found its epitope? At first sight it would appear that this could be a bit of a problem. As you can see from this figure, the part of the heavy chain that extends through the cell membrane into the interior of the cell is only a few amino acids in length -- way too short to do any signaling.

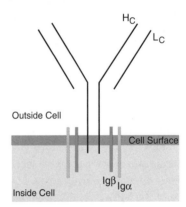

To make it possible for the external part of the BCR to signal what it has seen, B cells are equipped with two accessory proteins, Igα and Igβ, that associate with the Hc protein and protrude into the inside of the cell. Thus, the complete B cell receptor really has two parts: the Hc/Lc part outside the cell that recognizes the antigen but can't signal, and the Igα and Igβ proteins that can signal, but which are totally blind to what's going on outside the cell.

In order for a B cell to signal, many BCRs must be brought close together on the surface of the B cell. This clustering of BCRs can result when BCRs bind to an epitope that is repeated many times on a single antigen (e.g., a protein in which a sequence of amino acids is repeated many times).

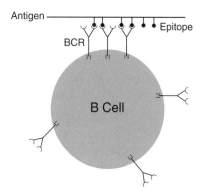

BCRs can also be clustered by binding to epitopes on antigens that are close together on the surface of an invader, or by binding to epitopes on antigens that are clumped together. Regardless of how it is accomplished, clustering or "crosslinking" of B cell receptors by antigen is essential for B cell activation. Here's why:

The tails of the Igα and Igβ signaling molecules interact with enzymes inside the cell, and when enough of these interactions are concentrated in one region, it sets off an enzymatic chain reaction that sends a message to the nucleus of the cell saying, "BCR engaged." So the trick to sending this message is to get lots of Igα and Igβ molecules together -- and that's exactly what clustering of B cell receptors does. The clustering of BCRs brings enough Igα and Igβ molecules together to set off the chain reaction that sends the signal. So BCR crosslinking is key.

You remember from the last lecture that fragments of complement proteins (e.g., C3b) can bind to (opsonize) invaders. This tag indicates that the invader has been recognized as dangerous by the innate immune system, and alerts innate system players like macrophages to destroy the opsonized invader. However, it turns out that antigens opsonsized by complement fragments can also alert the adaptive immune system. Here's how:

In addition to the B cell receptor and its associated signaling molecules, Igα and Igβ, there is another protein on the surface of the B cell that can play an important role in signaling. This protein is a receptor that can bind to complement fragments which are decorating an invader. Consequently, for an opsonized antigen, there are two receptors on a B cell that can bind the antigen: the BCR which recognizes an epitope on the antigen, and the complement receptor that recognizes the "decorations." When this happens, the

opsonized antigen acts as a "clamp" that brings the BCR and the complement receptor together on the surface of the B cell.

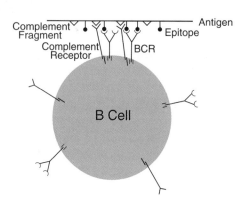

When the BCR and the complement receptor are "crosslinked" in this way by opsonized antigen, the signal that the BCR sends is greatly amplified. What this means in practice is that the number of BCRs that must be clustered to send the "receptor engaged" signal to the nucleus is decreased by at least 100-fold. Because the complement receptor can have such a dramatic effect on signaling, it is called a "co-receptor." The function of the co-receptor is especially important during the initial stages of an attack when the amount of antigen available to crosslink B cell receptors is limited. Recognition of opsonized invaders by the B cell co-receptor also serves to make B cells exquisitely sensitive to antigens that the innate system has identified as being dangerous. This is an excellent example of the "instructive" function of the innate system -- the decision on whether an invader is dangerous or not is generally made by the innate, not the adaptive, system.

HOW B CELLS ARE ACTIVATED

In order for B cells to produce antibodies, they must first be "activated." Roughly speaking, there are two ways this can be accomplished. One way definitely depends on T cell help. The other is called T cell-independent activation, but it is not clear exactly how independent of T cell help this activation pathway really is. When we talk about activation here, we are talking about activation of B cells that have never before encountered antigen. This kind of B cell is usually called a naive or virgin B cell. The rules for activating virgin B cells and for re-activating experienced B cells (those that have already encountered antigen) are somewhat different. For now we'll focus on virgin B cells that are recognizing their cognate antigens for the very first time.

T CELL-DEPENDENT ACTIVATION

T cell-dependent activation of a naive B cell requires two signals. The first is specific: recognition of cognate antigen by BCRs on the surface of the B cell, and the clustering of these BCRs and their associated signaling molecules. This clustering sends the "receptors engaged" message to the nucleus of the cell. However, this signal alone is not enough to activate the B cell -- a second signal is required. Immunologists call this the "co-stimulatory" signal, and it is usually provided by a helper T cell (Th cell). This is where the T cell-dependent part comes in. The most important co-stimulatory signal involves direct cell-cell contact between the B cell and the helper T cell. On the surfaces of activated Th cells are proteins called CD40L. When CD40L plugs into (ligates) a protein called CD40 on the surface of the B cell, a co-stimulatory signal is sent.

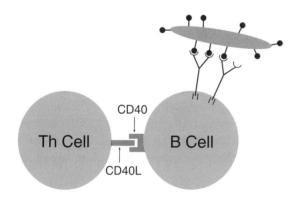

The interaction between these two proteins, CD40 and CD40L, is clearly very important for B cell activation -- humans who have a genetic defect in either of these proteins are unable to make a T cell-dependent antbody response.

Up until now, we have been talking about virgin B cells, but I need to say a few words about the activation requirements for experienced B cells. Once a B cell has been activated, it remembers that experience, and when it recognizes its cognate antigen again, the requirements for re-activation are less stringent than for the initial activation. How this memory works is not clear. The latest thinking is that re-activation definitely requires recognition of cognate antigen, but that in at least some cases, physical contact between B and Th cells is not necessary.

Now why would you want to have a system in which it is difficult to activate a B cell, and relatively easier to re-activate it? Well, one of the places you find a lot of experienced B cells is in the collection of memory cells that persists after your first exposure to an invader (e.g., the smallpox virus). These are "legit" B cells that have been through the stringent two-key selection for primary activation, and as a result are likely to be useful for protection against a second attack. In fact, these are the very B cells that you would like to activate quickly if you are attacked again. So making it easier for them to be re-activated makes perfect sense.

When B cells have been activated, they express new proteins on their surfaces. One of these is the receptor for IL-2, a growth factor that stimulates B cells to proliferate. So activation of B cells makes them able to receive cytokine signals that trigger proliferation. This coupling of activation to proliferation forms the basis for clonal selection -- only those B cells that have recognized their cognate antigen and have been activated (the selection part) will react to growth factors, proliferate, and form a clone of B cells with identical BCRs. The major supplier of growth factors like IL-2 is the helper T cell -- another reason T cell help is usually needed for B cell activation and proliferation.

T CELL-INDEPENDENT ACTIVATION OF B CELLS

In response to certain antigens, B cells can be activated with little or no T cell help. What these antigens have in common is that they are able to crosslink a ton of B cell receptors. In fact, clustering such a large number of BCRs appears to substitute for co-stimulation by CD40L. There are roughly two kinds of antigens that can do this. The first is an antigen that has repeated epitopes. A good example of this kind of antigen is a carbohydrate molecule of the type found on the surface of many bacterial cells. A carbohydrate molecule is made up of many repeating units, which, if recognized by the BCR as its cognate antigen, can bring many BCRs together and trigger activation. Of course, this type of activation is antigen specific: only those B cells whose receptors recognize the repeated epitope will be activated.

There is another, quite different way that B cells can be activated, independent of T cell help. In this case the antigen, usually called a "mitogen," binds to molecules on the B cell surface and clusters these molecules, dragging the BCRs along.

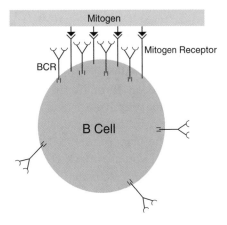

This "polyclonal activation" is independent of the specificity of the BCR -- the BCR just comes along for the ride. In this way, many different B cells with many different specificities can be activated by a single mitogen.

In the first lecture, I mentioned that two "keys" are required to activate the adaptive immune system. Just as with a safe deposit box, one of these keys is specific. For B cells, this specific key is the crosslinking of B cell receptors. The second key required for activation is nonspecific in that the same key works for all B cells. In the case of T cell-dependent activation, this key takes the form of the CD40L co-stimulatory molecule that plugs into the CD40 protein on the B cell surface. By making this "two key rule," a fail safe mechanism of activation is established in which the decision to activate is made by a "committee," not by just one cell.

But what about T cell-independent activation of B cells? Doesn't that violate the two-key rule for activation? We talked about crosslinking of the B cell receptors either by a specific antigen or by a mitogen, but where is the second key? This missing second key has bothered immunologists for some time, because it just seemed too dangerous for B cells to be activated simply by recognizing a target with repeated epitopes. So it was a great relief when it was recently discovered that T cell-independent activation really <u>does</u> require two keys!

In careful experiments, immunologists have now shown that when a B cell's receptors are crosslinked, the B cell begins to proliferate. However,

after it proliferates, the B cell won't secrete any antibodies -- not unless it receives a second signal. And what is this second key? For T cell-independent activation, the second key is a battle signal like the cytokine IFN-γ. What this means is that if a B cell recognizes a molecule with repeated epitopes like, for example, your own DNA, it may proliferate, but fortunately, no anti-DNA antibodies will be produced, because your immune system is not engaged in a battle with your own DNA. On the other hand, if the innate immune system is battling a bacterial invasion, and a B cell recognizes a carbohydrate antigen with repeated epitopes on the surface of a bacterial invader, that B cell will produce antibodies, because battle signals generated by the innate response will function as the second signal needed for complete B cell activation. So in response to T-cell independent antigens, B cells can take their cue directly from the innate immune system, and jump right into the battle without having to wait for T cells to be activated.

But there is something even more important going on here. Since T cells only recognize protein antigens, if all B cell activation required T cell help, the entire adaptive immune system would be focused only on proteins. This wouldn't be so great, since many of the most common invaders have carbohydrates or fats on their surfaces that are not found on the surfaces of human cells. Because these carbohydrates and fats are unique to invaders, they would make excellent targets for recognition by antibodies. So by allowing some antigens to activate B cells without T cell help, Mother Nature did a great thing: she increased the universe of antigens that the adaptive immune system can react against to include not only proteins, but carbohydrates and fats as well.

B CELL MATURATION

Once B cells have been activated, and have proliferated to build up their numbers, they are ready for the next stage in their life: maturation. Maturation can be divided roughly into three steps: isotype switching, in which the B cell decides which class of antibody it will produce; affinity maturation, in which the rearranged BCR undergoes mutation and selection that can lead to increased affinity for its cognate antigen; and a career decision, when the B cell decides whether to become an antibody factory (a plasma cell) or a memory B cell. The exact order of these maturation steps varies, and some B cells may skip one or more steps altogether.

ISOTYPE SWITCHING

After B cells are born in the bone marrow, they rearrange their gene segments for heavy and light chain (as we just discussed), and two classes of antibody molecules are displayed on their surfaces: IgM and IgD. These are the BCRs of the young B cell, and usually are called sIgM and sIgD, where the "s" stands for "surface." Interestingly, the same heavy chain mRNA is used to make both sIgM and sIgD, but the mRNA is spliced one way to yield an M-type constant region and another way to produce a D-type constant region. I haven't said much about IgD antibodies, because they represent only a tiny fraction of the circulating antibodies in a human, and it is unclear whether IgD antibodies actually perform any significant function. In contrast, sIgD, found on the surfaces of immature B cells, appears to serve important signaling functions during the maturation of B cells.

When a B cell exits the bone marrow, it doesn't secrete antibodies, because it hasn't been activated yet. This virgin B cell must first search for its cognate antigen. If the B cell finds it, <u>and</u> if it receives the co-stimulation it requires (that important second "key"), the B cell will be activated. Once activated, a B cell has the opportunity to change the class of antibody it makes from IgM to one of the other antibody isotypes: IgG, IgA, or IgE. The class of an antibody is determined by the constant region of its heavy chain, and located just next to the gene segment that encodes the constant region for IgM are the constant region segments for IgG, IgE, and IgA. So all the B cell has to do to change its isotype is to cut off the IgM constant region and paste on one of the other constant regions (deleting the DNA in between). Located between constant region segments on the chromosome are special switching signals that allow this cutting and pasting to take place. For example, here's what happens when a B cell switches from an IgM constant region to an IgG constant region:

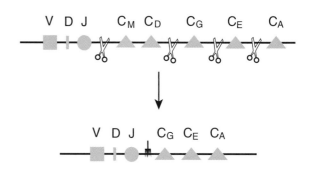

This choice of constant region segment (where to cut and paste) is not random: the cytokines that a B cell is "bathed" in at the time the switch takes place determine the B cell's choice of constant region. Since the different antibody classes that result from switching constant regions can perform different tasks, Mother Nature can insure that B cells produce antibodies appropriate to defend against different invaders simply by insuring that the appropriate cytokines are present when class switching takes place.

ANTIBODIES AND THEIR FUNCTIONS

Let's take a look at the four main classes of antibodies: IgM, IgA, IgG, and IgE. As you will see, because of the unique structure of its constant region, each class is particularly well suited to perform certain duties.

IgM Antibodies

When naive B cells are first activated, they mainly make IgM antibodies. You probably remember from the first lecture what an IgG antibody looks like:

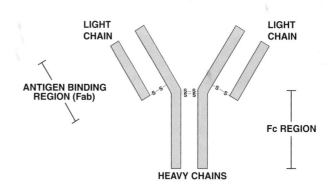

In contrast, an IgM antibody is like five IgG antibody molecules all stuck together. It's really massive!

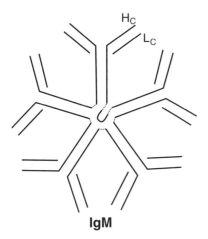

It turns out that producing this massive antibody early in infection is a great idea, because IgM antibodies are very good at activating the complement cascade (immunologists call this "fixing complement"). Here's how it works:

Some of the complement proteins (about thirty of them!) form a big complex called C1. Despite its size, this complex of proteins cannot activate the complement cascade, because it's bound to an inhibitor molecule. However, if two or more C1 complexes are brought close together, their inhibitors fall off, and the C1 molecules can initiate a cascade of events that produces a C3 convertase. Now we're in business, because, as you remember from the last lecture, the C3 convertase converts C3 to C3b, setting up an amplification loop that produces more and more C3b. So the trick to activating complement by this "classical" pathway is to bring two or more molecules of C1 together -- and IgM does just that. When IgM antibodies bind to an invader, C1 complexes can bind to the Fc regions of the IgM antibodies. Now, each IgM antibody has five Fc regions close together (this is the important point), so if two C1 complexes bind to the Fc regions of the same IgM antibody, they will be close enough together to set off the complement cascade. So the bottom line is: The IgM antibody binds to the invader, recruits C1 molecules to the scene, and sets off the complement chain reaction.

This is a nice example of the innate immune system (complement) cooperating with the adaptive immune system (IgM antibodies) to destroy an invader. In fact, the term "complement" was coined by immunologists when they first discovered that antibodies were much more effective in dealing with invaders if they were "complemented" by other proteins -- the complement proteins. The alternative (spontaneous) complement activation pathway that we talked about in the last lecture is totally non-specific: Any unprotected surface is fair game. In contrast, the classical (antibody-dependent) activation pathway is quite specific: Only those antigens to which antibodies bind will be targeted for complement attack.

Some IgG antibodies can also "fix" complement, because C1 can bind to the Fc region of certain subclasses of IgG. However, IgG antibodies are real wimps with only one Fc region per molecule. So to bring two C1 complexes close enough together to get things started requires that two molecules of IgG bind very close together on the surface of the invading pathogen -- and this is only likely to happen when there is a lot of IgG around. So early in an infection, when antibodies are just beginning to be made, IgM antibodies have a great advantage over IgG antibodies, because they fix complement so efficiently. In addition, IgM antibodies are very good at "neutralizing" viruses by binding to them and preventing them from docking on cells they would like to infect. So IgM is a good "first antibody" to defend against viral or bacterial infections.

IgA Antibodies

Here's a question for you: What is the most abundant antibody class in the human body? No, it's not IgG. It's IgA! This is really a trick question, because I told you earlier that IgG was the most abundant antibody class in the blood -- which is true. It turns out, however, that we humans synthesize more IgA antibodies than all other antibodies combined. Why so much IgA? Because IgA is the main antibody class that guards the mucosal surfaces of the body, and a human has about 400 square meters of mucosal surfaces to defend. So although there aren't a lot of IgA antibodies circulating in the blood, there are tons of them in the mucosal surfaces. One reason IgA antibodies are so good at defending against invaders that would like to penetrate the mucosal barrier is that IgA molecules are like two IgG molecules held together by a "clip." Each IgG molecule has two antigen binding regions (two "hands"), so the "dimeric" IgA molecule has <u>four</u> hands to bind to pathogens.

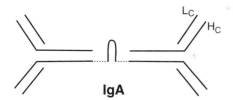

IgA

Because of its four antigen-binding regions, IgA is very good at collecting pathogens together into clumps that are large enough to be swept out of the body with the mucus.

IgA has another interesting function: It is secreted into the milk of nursing mothers. This makes sense, because many of the pathogens that babies encounter are taken in through their mouths -- babies like to put their mouths on everything. The IgA in mother's milk coats the baby's intestinal mucosa and provides protection against pathogens that the baby ingests. Although IgA antibodies are great against mucosal invaders, they are totally useless at fixing complement, because C1 won't bind to the IgA antibodies' Fc region.

IgG Antibodies

IgG antibodies (sometimes called gamma globulins) come in a number of different subclasses with different functions. For example, the IgG1 subclass is very good at binding to invaders to opsonize them for ingestion by professional phagocytes. This is because macrophages and neutrophils have receptors on their surfaces that can bind to the Fc portion of IgG1 antibodies.

Another subclass of IgG antibodies, IgG3, fixes complement better than any other IgG subclass. In addition, natural killer cells have receptors on their surfaces that can bind to the Fc region of IgG3. As a result, IgG3 can bind to a target cell (e.g., a virus-infected cell) with its Fab region, and form a bridge between the target cell and the NK cell with its Fc region. Not only does this bring the NK cell close to its target, but having its Fc receptors bound actually stimulates an NK cell to be a more effective killer. This process is called "antibody-dependent cellular cytotoxicity" (ADCC) -- the NK cell does the killing, but the antibody provides the specificity.

IgG antibodies are also good at neutralizing viruses by binding to the region of the virus that nor-mally would attach to its target cell. Finally, IgG antibodies from the mother's blood are able to cross the placenta and enter the circulation of the fetus. This provides the fetus with a supply of IgG antibodies to tide it over until it begins to produce its own -- several months after birth.

IgE Antibodies

The IgE antibody class has an interesting history. In the early 1900's, a French physician named Charles Richet was sailing with Prince Albert of Monaco (Grace Kelly's father-in-law). The prince remarked to Richet that it was very strange how some people reacted violently to the sting of the Portuguese Man of War, and he suggested that this phenomenon might be worthy of study. Richet took his advice, and when he returned to Paris, he decided, as a first experiment, to test how much Man of War toxin was required to kill a dog. Don't ask me why he decided to use dogs in his experiments. Maybe there were lots of stray dogs around back then, or perhaps he just didn't like mice. Anyway, the experiment was a success and he was able to determine the amount of toxin that was lethal. However, many of the dogs he used in this first experiment survived, because they didn't receive the lethal dose. Not being the kind of guy who would waste a good dog, Richet decided to inject these leftover dogs again with the toxin to see what would happen. His expectation was that these dogs might have become immune to the effects of the toxin, and that the first injection would have provided protection (prophylaxis) against a second injection. You can imagine his surprise then, when all the dogs died -- even the ones that received tiny amounts of toxin in the second injection! Since the first injection had the opposite effect of protection, Richet coined the word "anaphylaxis" to describe this phenomenon ("ana" is a prefix meaning "opposite"). Richet continued these studies on anaphylactic shock, and in 1913, he received the Nobel Prize for his work. One lesson here is that if a prince suggests you study something, you should take his advice seriously!

Immunologists now know that anaphylactic shock is caused by mast cells degranulating. Mast cells are white blood cells that are involved in protecting us against parasitic infections. Inside mast cells are lots of granules that contain all kinds of pharmacologically-active chemicals, the most famous of which is histamine. When the mast cell encounters a parasite, it dumps the contents of these granules onto the parasite to kill it. In addition to killing parasites, mast cell degranulation can also cause an allergic reaction, and in extreme cases, anaphylactic shock. Here's how it works:

On the first exposure to the allergen (e.g., the Man of War toxin), some people (and dogs), for reasons that are far from clear, make lots of IgE antibodies directed against the allergen. Mast cells have receptors on their surfaces that can bind to the Fc region of IgE antibodies.

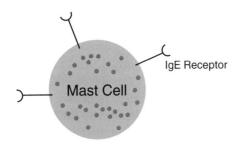

BEFORE EXPOSURE

When these receptors bind IgE antibodies, the mast cell is like a grenade waiting to explode.

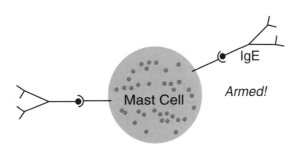

AFTER FIRST EXPOSURE

On the second exposure to the allergen, those IgE molecules that are already bound to the surface of the mast cell now can bind to the allergen. Because allergens are usually small proteins with a repeating sequence, the allergen can crosslink the IgE molecules on the mast cell surface, dragging the Fc receptors

together. This clustering of Fc receptors is similar to the crosslinking of B cell receptors in that it results in a signal being sent. However, in this case, the signal says "degranulate," and the mast cell dumps its granules into your tissues.

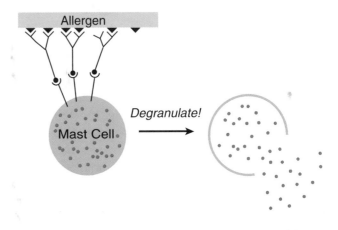

Histamines and other chemicals released from mast cell granules increase capillary permeability, so that fluid escapes from the capillaries into the tissues -- that's why you get a runny nose and watery eyes when you have an allergic reaction. This is usually a rather local effect, but if the toxin spreads throughout the body and triggers massive degranulation of mast cells, things can get very serious. In such a case, the release of fluid from the blood into tissues can reduce the blood volume so much that the heart no longer can pump efficiently, resulting in a heart attack. In addition, histamine from the granules can cause smooth muscles around the windpipe to contract, making it difficult to breathe. In extreme cases, this contraction can be strong enough to cause suffocation. Here in Colorado we don't worry much about Portuguese Men of War, but we are concerned about bees, because the toxin in a bee sting can cause fatal anaphylactic shock in some individuals.

This brings us to an interesting question: Why are B cells allowed to switch the class of antibody they make anyway? Wouldn't it be safer just to stick with good old IgM antibodies? Well, let's suppose you have a respiratory infection like the common cold. Would you want to be stuck making only IgM antibodies? Certainly not. You'd want lots of IgA antibodies to be secreted into the mucosa that line your respiratory tract. On the other hand, if you have a parasitic infection (say, some sort of worms), you'd want IgE antibodies to be produced, because IgE antibodies can cause mast cells to degranulate and kill those worms. The beauty of this system is that the different classes of antibodies are uniquely suited to defend against certain invaders.

ANTIBODY CLASS	ANTIBODY PROPERTIES
IgM	Great Complement Fixer Good Opsonizer First Antibody Made
IgA	Resistant to Stomach Acid Protects Mucosal Surfaces Secreted in Milk
IgG	OK Complement Fixer Good Opsonizer Helps NK Cells Kill (ADCC) Can Cross Placenta
IgE	Defends Against Parasites Causes Anaphylactic Shock Causes Allergies

Now suppose that Mother Nature could arrange to have your immune system make IgA antibodies when you have a cold, and IgE antibodies when you have a parasitic infection. Wouldn't that be neat? Well, it turns out that this is exactly what happens! Here's how it works:

The isotype switch is controlled by the cytokines that B cells encounter when class switching takes place, and certain cytokines or combinations of cytokines influence B cells to switch to one isotype or another. For example, if B cells switch in an environment that is rich in IL-4 and IL-5, they preferentially switch their isotype (class) from IgM to IgE -- just right for worms. On the other hand, if there is a lot of IFN-γ around, B cells switch to produce IgG3 antibodies that work great against bacteria and viruses. Or, if a cytokine called TGF-β is present during the class switch, B cells preferentially change from IgM to IgA production -- perfect for the common cold.

So in order to make the right antibody response to a given invader, all Mother Nature has to do is to arrange to have the right cytokines present when B cells switch isotypes. But how could this be accomplished? Well, you remember that helper T cells are "quarterback" cells that direct the immune response. One way they do this is by producing cytokines that influence B cells to make antibodies that are appropriate for a given invader. To learn how Th cells know which cytokines to make, you'll have to wait for the next lectures when we discuss antigen presentation and T cell activation. But I'll tell you now that the cytokines made by Th cells, and the ability of B cells to switch from producing IgM to producing one of the other antibody classes make it possible for the adaptive immune system to respond with antibodies tailor-made for each kind of invader -- be it a bacterium, a flu virus, or a worm. What could be better than that!

SOMATIC HYPERMUTATION

As if class switching weren't neat enough, there is yet another great thing that can happen to B cells as they mature -- somatic hypermutation. Normally, the overall mutation rate of DNA in mammalian cells is extremely low, about one mutated base per trillion bases per DNA replication cycle. It has to be this low or we'd all end up looking like Star Wars characters with three eyes and six ears. However, in very restricted regions of the chromosomes of B cells -- those regions that contain the V, D, and J segments that encode the antibody heavy and light chains -- an extremely high rate of mutation can take place. In these regions, mutation rates as high as one mutated base per thousand bases per generation have been measured. We're talking serious mutations here! This high rate of mutation is called somatic hypermutation, and it occurs after the V, D, and J segments have been selected, and usually after class switching has taken place. So hypermutation is a relatively late event in the maturation of B cells, and B cells that still make IgM antibodies usually have not undergone somatic hypermutation.

Somatic hypermutation changes (mutates) the part of the rearranged antibody gene that encodes the antigen binding region of the antibody. Depending on the mutation, there are three possible outcomes: the affinity of the antibody molecule for its cognate antigen may remain unchanged, or it may be increased, or it may be decreased. Now comes the neat part. It turns out that for these maturing B cells to continue to proliferate, they must be continually re-stimulated by binding to their cognate antigen. Therefore, those B cells whose BCRs have mutated to a higher affinity are stimulated more often (because their BCRs bind better), and as a result, they proliferate more than B cells with lower affinity receptors. So by using somatic hypermutation to make changes in the BCR, and by using binding and proliferation to select those mutations that have increased the BCR's ability to bind to antigen, B cell receptors can be "fine tuned." The result is a collection of B cells whose receptors have a higher average affinity for their cognate antigen. This process is called affinity maturation.

By going through the processes of class switching and affinity maturation, B cells can change both their Fc region (by class switching) and their Fab region (by somatic hypermutation). Both changes take place in secondary lymphoid organs like the lymph nodes, both changes are driven by cytokines that are provided mainly by helper T cells, and both changes result in B cells that are better adapted to deal with invaders.

B CELLS MAKE A CAREER CHOICE

The final step in the maturation of a B cell is the choice of profession. This can't be too tough, because a B cell really has only two fates to choose between: to become a plasma cell or a memory cell. Plasma cells are antibody factories. If a B cell chooses to become a plasma cell, it usually travels to the spleen or back to the bone marrow, and begins to produce the secreted form of the BCR -- the antibody molecule. Plasma B cells crank out about two thousand of these antibodies each second, and as a result of this heroic effort, most plasma B cells live only a few days. The details of how a B cell decides to become either a memory or a plasma cell are still not understood. However, the latest thinking is that becoming a plasma cell is usually the default option, and that to avoid this fate, a B cell must receive additional stimulation, probably involving repeated ligation of its CD40 protein by CD40L on the surface of a helper T cell.

Although the choice to become a memory B cell is not quite so dramatic as the decision to become a plasma cell, it is extremely important, for it is the memory B cell that remembers your first exposure to a pathogen, and defends you against subsequent exposures. Memory B cells usually have undergone class switching, so their constant region is appropriate to defend against the invader they remember. In addition, most memory cells have experienced somatic hypermutation, so they have high affinity BCRs that can respond more easily to the low levels of antigen that are present at the beginning of an infection. Further, memory B cells have reduced requirements for activation relative to naive B cells. In short, memory B cells are "ready to go" to defend against a second attack.

It is clear that memory B cells can confer lifelong immunity to infection. For example, in 1781 Swedish traders brought the measles virus to the isolated Faeroe islands. In 1846, when another ship carrying sailors infected with measles visited the islands, people who were older than sixty-four years did not contract the disease -- they still had antibodies against the measles virus. How this long-lasting B cell immunity is maintained is currently under debate. Even the longest-lived antibodies (the IgG class) only survive for about a month, so antibodies must be made continuously to provide long-lasting protection. Some evidence suggests that memory B cells can live a long time. Other experiments indicate that memory B cells are short lived, but that they periodically proliferate when they are re-stimulated by exposure to antigen. This could be antigen that is left around after the attack, or it might be another antigen that is similar enough to the invader to re-stimulate memory B cells. According to this scenario, it would actually be the descendants of the original memory B cells that make the antibodies which confer immunity. Hopefully, the mechanism(s) for the maintenance of memory will soon be understood, for this information would be of great value in designing effective vaccines.

SUMMARY FIGURE

Our summary figure now includes the innate immune system from the last lecture, plus the B cells and antibodies that we talked about today.

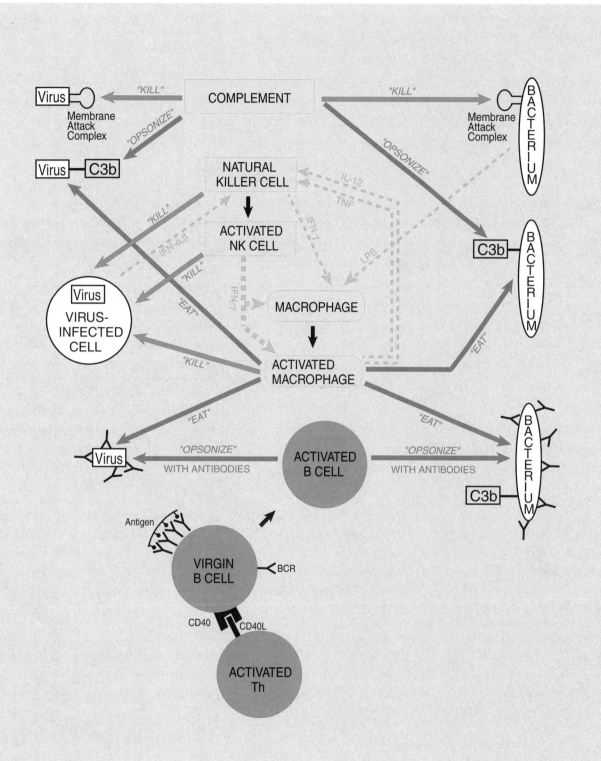

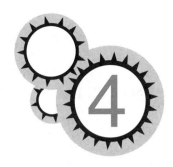

4

MHC MOLECULES AND ANTIGEN PRESENTATION

REVIEW

In the last lecture we discussed B cells and antibodies, so let's do a bit of review. We talked about how the B cell receptor (BCR), which is responsible for recognizing what is happening outside the B cell, actually has two parts: a recognition part (made up of the heavy and light chain proteins), and a signaling part (made up of two proteins, Igα and Igβ). The final genes that encode the heavy and light chains are made by selecting gene segments in a high stakes "card game." The result is a collection of B cells with receptors so diverse that they can probably recognize any organic molecule in the universe.

Signaling by B cell receptors requires that multiple BCRs be clustered (crosslinked). When the antigen binding regions of the light and heavy chains (the parts of the BCR that are responsible for antigen recognition) are crosslinked, the Igα and Igβ signaling molecules that are associated with the heavy chains are dragged close together. When enough Igα and Igβ molecules are clustered in this way, a threshold amount of enzymatic activity is reached, and the "receptor engaged" signal is sent to the nucleus of the B cell.

Activation of a B cell requires two "keys," and crosslinking of B cell receptors is the first key. There are two ways that the second, "co-stimulatory" key can be provided. The first depends on helper T cells, so this type of activation is called T cell dependent. One co-stimulatory signal that appears to be absolutely required for helper T cells to activate inexperienced B cells is an interaction between the CD40 protein on the surface of the B cell and a molecule called CD40 ligand on the surface of a Th cell. Thus, co-stimulation of virgin B cells by Th cells requires that these two cells make physical contact.

B cells can also be activated without T cell help, and there are two ways that this can be accomplished. First, B cell receptors can be crosslinked by antigen that has repeated epitopes. In this case, only B cells whose BCRs bind to the repeated epitope are activated, so activation is specific to that particular antigen. In a second scenario, large numbers of B cells can be activated by molecules called mitogens. These mitogens cause BCRs to cluster together, not by interacting with the BCR itself, but rather by binding to other molecules on the B cell surface which can then drag the BCRs together. As a result, mitogens can activate B cells without regard to the specificity of their B cell receptors.

A key feature of both modes of T cell-independent activation is that a very large number of B cell receptors must be crosslinked. This high level of crosslinking appears to at least partially substitute for the CD40L co-stimulatory signal that is provided by Th cells during T cell-dependent activation. I say "partially substitute" because immunologists now realize that although crosslinking a ton of BCRs is required for T cell-independent activation of B cells, it is not enough. For full activation, a second signal is required, and this signal can be supplied by the innate system in the form of "battle cytokines." Thus, activation of a virgin B cell always requires two signals: crosslinking of BCRs, and a "danger" signal provided either by a Th cell that has been activated in response to an invasion or by the innate system engaged in battle.

After B cells are activated, they begin to mature. During B cell maturation, two very interesting things can happen: class switching and somatic hypermutation. The default option for B cells is the production of IgM antibodies, so these are the first antibodies produced in response to a pathogen that has not been encountered before. However, as a B cell matures, it can choose another kind of constant region for its heavy chain molecules, so that antibodies of the IgG, IgA, or IgE class can be produced. This class (isotype) switching does not change the antigen binding region (Fab) of the antibody, so the antibody recognizes the same antigen before and after its class has been switched. What changes is the Fc region of the heavy chain (the "legs," if you will), and it is this part of the antibody that determines how the antibody functions. The choice of antibody class is determined by the cytokines that are present in the local environment of the B cell when the class switch takes place. Thus, by arranging to have appropriate cytokines produced at the appropriate places, Mother Nature can insure that the antibodies produced will be just right to defend against a particular invader.

The other change that can take place as a B cell matures is somatic hypermutation. In contrast to class switching in which the Fc region changes, somatic hypermutation alters the part of the antibody that binds to antigen (the Fab or "hands" region). Since the probability of a B cell being triggered to proliferate depends on the affinity of its BCR for antigen, those B cells in which somatic hypermutation has increased the binding affinity will proliferate most. As a result of this process of somatic hypermutation and proliferation, a collection of B cells will emerge that has high affinity BCRs which bind very tightly to antigen. These cells are especially useful as memory B cells, because their affinity-matured BCRs allow them to be reactivated early in a second infection while the number of invaders is still relatively small.

It is important to note that although B cells can be activated with or without T cell help, the outcomes in these two cases are very different. T cell-independent activation usually results in the production of IgM antibodies. In contrast, T cell-dependent activation usually produces affinity-matured, IgG, IgA or IgE antibodies. One reason for this difference is that class switching and somatic hypermutation are both cytokine driven, and Th cells are the major sources of these cytokines. Moreover, both processes probably require ligation of CD40 on B cells by CD40L -- and this proteins is expressed on activated Th cells.

As B cells mature, they must also decide whether to become short-lived plasma cells that make lots of the secreted form of the BCR that we call antibodies, or to go back to the resting state as longer-lived, memory B cells. Exactly how this decision is made is not clear, but it is suspected that T cell help is required to produce memory B cells.

MHC PROTEINS AND ANTIGEN PRESENTATION

You recall from the first lecture that to be activated, a T cell must recognize its cognate antigen presented by an MHC molecule on the surface of an antigen presenting cell. In this lecture, we'll look more closely at these MHC proteins, and examine how antigens are prepared for presentation. Finally, we'll discuss those cells that specialize in presenting antigen -- the professional antigen presenting cells or "APCs."

CLASS I MHC MOLECULES

The crystal structures of both class I and class II MHC molecules have now been solved, so we have a pretty good idea of what both molecules look like. The class I molecule has a peptide binding groove that is closed at both ends, so the "hotdog must fit the bun." When immunologists pried peptides from the grasp of class I molecules and sequenced them, they found that most of them are eight to eleven amino acids in length. These peptides are anchored at the ends, so the variation in length is accommodated by letting the peptide bulge out a bit in the center.

Each human has three genes for MHC I molecules (called HLA-A, HLA-B, and HLA-C), located on chromosome six. Because we have two chromosome sixes (one from Mom and one from Dad), we each have a total of six MHC I genes. In the human population, there are many different forms of the three MHC I molecules. For example, there are at least sixty different forms of the HLA-A molecule. All of these have the same rough shape (e.g., they all have a binding groove), but they differ from one another by one or a few amino acids. Immunologists call molecules that have many forms "polymorphic." In contrast, the β2-microglobulin protein, which goes together with the proteins encoded by the HLA-A, HLA-B, or HLA-C genes to make up the final MHC I molecule, is "monomorphic" -- all of us have the same β2-microglobulin protein.

Because they are polymorphic, MHC I molecules can have different binding motifs, and therefore can present peptides that have different kinds of amino acids at their ends. Some MHC I molecules, for example, bind to peptides that have hydrophobic amino acids at one end, whereas other MHC molecules prefer basic amino acids at this anchor position. Because humans have the possibility of expressing up to six different class I molecules, each of us will have class I molecules that can present peptides with a range of binding motifs. Moreover, although MHC I molecules are quite picky about binding to certain amino acids at the ends of the peptide, they are quite promiscuous in their selection of amino acids at the center of the peptide. As a result, a given MHC I molecule can bind to and present a large number of different peptides, all of which have a particular binding motif at their ends.

CLASS II MHC MOLECULES

In contrast to class I molecules, the class II binding groove is open at both ends, so the "hotdog can hang out of the bun." As you might expect from this feature, peptides that bind to class II molecules are longer than those that occupy the closed groove of class I molecules -- in the range of thirteen to twenty-five amino acids. Further, for class II, the critical amino acids that anchor the peptides are spaced along the binding groove instead of being clustered at the ends. These features suggest that the enzymes which generate peptides suitable for class I presentation are probably quite different from those that generate class II peptides. Like those of class I, class II MHC molecules are very polymorphic, with lots of different forms represented in the general population.

ANTIGEN PRESENTATION BY CLASS I MHC MOLECULES

MHC I molecules are "billboards" that display fragments of proteins manufactured by the cell. Immunologists call these "endogenous" proteins. These include ordinary cellular proteins like enzymes and structural proteins as well as proteins encoded by viruses and other parasites that infect the cell. For example, when a virus enters a cell, it takes over the cellular biosynthetic machinery, and uses it to produce proteins encoded by viral genes. These viral proteins are displayed by class I MHC molecules along with all the normal cellular proteins. So in effect, the MHC I billboard displays a "sampling" of all the proteins that are being made inside the cell. Almost every cell in the human body expresses class I molecules on its surface, although the number of molecules vary from cell to cell.

As a result, almost every cell is an "open book" that can be checked by T cells to be sure it has not been invaded by a virus or other parasite.

The way endogenous proteins are processed and loaded onto MHC I molecules is very interesting. As you probably know, mRNA is translated into protein in the cytoplasm of the cell. Most of the time, this process goes quite nicely, but sometimes mistakes are made, and the proteins produced don't fold up quite right. Also, as a result of normal wear and tear, some proteins get damaged. To make sure cells don't fill up with defective proteins, old or useless proteins are fed into protein-destroying "machines" in the cytoplasm that function rather like wood chippers. These protein chippers are called proteasomes, and they cut proteins up into small pieces (peptides). Most of these peptides are then broken down further into individual amino acids which are re-used to make new proteins. However, some of the peptides created by the proteasomes are carried by specific transporter proteins (TAP1 and TAP2) across the membrane of the endoplasmic reticulum (ER) -- a large sack-like structure inside the cell from which most proteins destined for transport to the cell surface begin their journey.

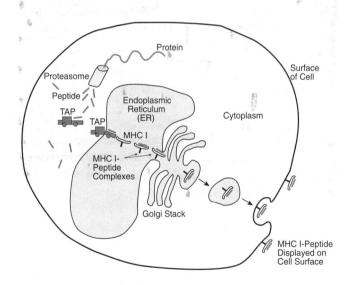

Once inside the ER, some of these peptides are chosen to be loaded into the groove of MHC I molecules. I say "chosen," because, as we discussed, not all peptides will fit into the groove of a class I MHC molecule. For starters, a peptide must be the right length -- about nine amino acids. In addition, the amino acids at the ends of the peptide must be compatible with the anchor amino acids that line the ends of the groove of the MHC molecule. Obviously, not all of the "chips" prepared by the proteasome will be proper, and those that are not are shipped back out of the ER into the cytoplasm to be broken down further. Once MHC I molecules are loaded with peptides, they proceed to the surface of the cell for display.

Now, as you could see from the last figure, there are three main processes involved in the MHC I display of peptides: generation of the peptide by the proteasome, transport of the peptide into the ER by the TAP transporter, and binding of the peptide to the groove of the MHC I molecule. A lot of mystery still surrounds these processes, but I'll tell you about some of the recent discoveries that shed light on how this all works.

In "ordinary" cells like liver cells and heart cells, the function of proteasomes is to deal with defective proteins, so as you can imagine, the chippers are not too particular about how the proteins are cut up -- they just hack away. As a result, some of the peptides will be appropriate for MHC presentation, but most will not. In contrast, in cells like macrophages that specialize in presenting antigen, this chipping is not so random. For example, binding of IFN-γ to receptors on the surface of a macrophage upregulates expression of proteins called LMP. These LMP proteins replace normal subunits of the proteasomes, and customize the proteasomes so that they preferentially cut proteins after hydrophobic or basic amino acids. Why, you ask? Because the TAP transporter and MHC I molecules both favor peptides that have either hydrophobic or basic C-termini. So in APCs, LMP proteins modify standard proteasomes so they will produce custom-made peptides for class I presentation, thereby increasing the efficiency of class I display.

Proteasomes are also not too particular about the size of peptides they make, and since the magic number for class I presentation is about nine amino acids, you might imagine that the ER would be flooded with useless peptides that were either too long or too short. However, it turns out that the TAP transporter has the highest affinity for peptides that are between about eight and thirteen amino acids long. Therefore, the TAP transporter screens peptides produced by proteasomes, and preferentially transports those that have the right kinds of C-termini and which are approximately the right length for binding to MHC I molecules.

ANTIGEN PRESENTATION BY CLASS II MHC MOLECULES

In contrast to class I MHC molecules, which are expressed on almost every kind of cell, class II molecules are expressed exclusively on cells of the immune system. This makes sense, because class I molecules specialize in presenting proteins that are manufactured inside the cell (endogenous proteins), and this gives killer T cells a chance to check most cells in the body for viral or other infections. On the other hand, class II MHC molecules function as billboards that display what is happening outside the cell, so that helper T cells can be alerted to danger. Therefore, relatively few cells expressing class II are required for this task -- just enough to sample the environment in various parts of the body.

The two proteins that make up the MHC II molecule (called α and β chains) are produced in the cytoplasm and are injected into the endoplasmic reticulum where they bind to a third protein called the invariant chain. This invariant chain performs several functions. First, it sits in the groove of the MHC II molecule and keeps it from picking up other peptides in the ER. This is important, because the ER is full of endogenous peptides that have been processed by proteasomes for loading onto class I MHC molecules. If these fragments of endogenous proteins were loaded onto class II molecules, then MHC class I and class II would both display the same kind of peptides: those made from proteins produced in the cell. Since the goal is to have MHC II molecules present antigens that come from outside the cell, the invariant chain performs an important function by acting as a "chaperone" that makes sure "inappropriate suitors" (endogenous peptides) don't get picked up by MHC II molecules in the ER.

The invariant chain's second function is to guide class II MHC molecules out through the Golgi stack to a special vesicle in the cytoplasm called an endosome. When biologists don't understand something very well, they usually call it a "-some" -- a suffix that means "body." So it makes sense that the place where peptides are loaded onto class II MHC molecules is called an endosome, because very little is known for certain about what goes on there. The current thinking is that under the guidance of the invariant chain, MHC II molecules make their way from the ER to the endosome. Meanwhile, proteins that are hanging around outside the cell (exogenous proteins) are taken inside

＊ LMP encoded for in genes adjacent to those for TAP in MHC gene
Role is not clear yet ∴ some cells deficient in
the expression of these proteasome subunits are capable of
processing Ag and delivering it to Class I molecules in op.

the cell, and enclosed in a vesicle called a phagosome. This phagosome then merges with the endosome, and enzymes in the endosome chop up the exogenous proteins from the phagosome into small peptides. Then the part of the invariant chain that is guarding the groove of the MHC molecule is displaced, and an exogenous peptide is loaded into the empty groove of the MHC II molecule. Finally, the complex of MHC II plus peptide is transported to the cell surface for display.

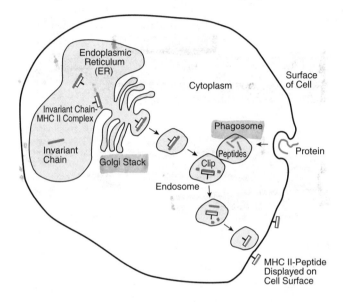

This is probably more or less what happens, but the details are still fuzzy. The important point, however, is that Mother Nature has arranged two separate loading sites and pathways for MHC I and II. It is this separation of loading sites and pathways that allows the class I billboard to advertize what's going on inside the cell (for CTLs), and the class II billboard to advertize what's happening outside (for Th cells).

MHC PROTEINS AND ORGAN TRANSPLANTS

Studies on organ and tissue transplantation actually began in the 1930's with experiments involving mouse tumors. In those days, tumors were usually induced by rubbing some horrible chemical on the skin of a mouse, and then waiting for a long time for a tumor to develop. Because it was so much trouble to make these tumors, biologists wanted to keep the tumors alive for study after the mouse had died, and they did this by injecting some of the tumor cells into

another, healthy mouse where the tumor cells would continue to grow. What they observed, however, was that the tumor cells could only be successfully transplanted when the two mice were from a strain of mice in which there had been a lot of inbreeding. The more inbred the strain, the better the chance for survival of the transplant. This provided the impetus for the creation of a number of inbred mouse strains that immunologists depend on today. Just so you know, it takes over two years of constant breeding to produce a strain of mice that is truly inbred -- a strain in which all the mice have the same genetic makeup.

Once inbred mouse strains were available, immunologists began to study the transplantation of normal tissues from one mouse to another. What they observed right away was that if a small patch of skin from one mouse (the donor) was grafted onto the skin of another mouse (the recipient) this new skin retained its healthy pink color and continued to grow so long as the two mice were from the same inbred strain. In contrast, when this experiment was tried with mice that were not inbred, the transplanted skin turned white within hours (suggesting the blood supply had been cut off) and invariably died. Immunologists figured this immediate graft rejection must be due to some genetic incompatibility, because it did not occur with inbred mice that have the same genes, so they set about to identify the genes that are involved in "tissue compatibility" (histocompatibility). To accomplish this, they bred mice to create strains that differed by only a few genes, yet which still were incompatible for tissue transplants. Whenever they did these experiments, they kept identifying genes that were grouped in a complex on mouse chromosome seventeen -- a complex they eventually called the "major histocompatibility complex" or MHC.

So the MHC molecules that we have been discussing in the context of antigen presentation are the very molecules that are responsible for immediate rejection of transplanted organs. It turns out that CTLs are particularly sensitive to MHC molecules that are "foreign," and when they see them, they attack and kill the cells that express them. One of their favorite targets are the cells that make up the blood vessels that are part of the donor organ. By destroying these vessels, CTLs cut off the blood supply to the transplanted organ, usually resulting in its death. It is for this reason that transplant surgeons try to match donors and recipients that have the same MHC molecules.

THE LOGIC OF MHC PRESENTATION

Now let me ask you a few questions to see if you've been following what I've been saying. Why do you think Mother Nature made MHC molecules so polymorphic? After all, there are so many different forms in the population that most of us inherit genes for six different class I molecules. Doesn't this seem a little excessive? I mean, why not just have everybody express one MHC I molecule? That would certainly make things a lot simpler for transplant surgeons.

Suppose, however, that we all did have just one gene for MHC I molecules, and that it was the same for everyone. Now suppose a virus were to mutate so that none of its viral peptides could be processed, transported, and bound to that MHC I molecule? Such a virus could wipe out the whole human population, because no T cells could be activated to destroy virus-infected cells. So polymorphic MHC molecules give at least some people in the population a chance of surviving an attack by a clever pathogen.

Okay, so if having six MHC I molecules is good, wouldn't 1,000 be better? Why not 10,000? After all, Mother Nature certainly could have arranged to make our MHC molecules as diverse as the B and T cell receptors, just by using the strategy of mixing and matching gene segments. But she didn't do this -- and for a very good reason. The T cell receptor must recognize not only its cognate peptide presented by the MHC molecule but also the MHC molecule itself (more about this "dual recognition" next lecture). For a virgin T cell to be activated, about 100 of its T cell receptors must recognize a particular MHC molecule with its associated peptide. So if each antigen presenting cell expressed 1,000 different MHC molecules, there would be too few of any one kind of MHC molecule presenting a given antigen to efficiently activate a T cell. No, I don't know why she picked six! I guess it must have been a good compromise.

Another interesting question is: Why bother with MHC presentation at all? Why not just let T cells recognize un-presented antigen the way B cells do? This is really a two-part question, since we are talking about two rather different displays: class I and class II. So let's take them one at a time.

Clearly, one reason for class I presentation is to focus the attention of killer T cells on virus-infected cells, not on free virus. First, it would be way too "expensive" to use CTLs to deal with free virus. Each plasma B cell can pump out about 10,000 antibody molecules per second, and these antibodies can tag free virus for destruction by professional phagocytes, and can bind to viruses to keep them from infecting cells. So antibodies are cheap and effective weapons for use against free virus. In contrast, CTLs are expensive, high-tech weapons specifically designed to deal with infected cells -- and class I display lets the CTL look into a cell to determine whether it is a suitable target. Second, it would be way too dangerous to have un-presented antigen signal T cell killing. Imagine how terrible it would be if uninfected cells happened to have debris from dead viruses stuck to their surfaces, and killer T cells recognized this un-presented antigen and killed these "innocent bystander" cells. That certainly wouldn't do.

There's another reason why class I display is so important. Most viral proteins never make their way to the surface of an infected cell where a CTL could see them, so without class I display, many virus-infected cells would go undetected. In fact, one of the real beauties of MHC I display is that, in principle, all viral proteins can be chopped up into peptides and displayed by MHC class I on the surface of a virus-infected cell. This gives the CTL lots more targets. When you think of it, B cells are really at a disadvantage because they recognize "native" antigen that has not been chopped up and presented. Most proteins must be folded in order to function properly, and as a result of this folding, many targets (epitopes) that a B cell might recognize are unavailable for viewing, because they are on the inside of a folded protein molecule. In contrast, when a protein is chopped up into short peptides and presented by MHC I molecules, these targets can't hide from a T cell.

So MHC class I presentation makes a lot of sense, but what about class II presentation? Couldn't helper T cells just recognize free antigen? After all, they aren't killers, so there isn't the problem of bystander killing. That's true, of course, but there is a safety issue. Helper T cells require APCs to present them with antigen, and these APCs don't present antigen efficiently unless a battle is raging. As a result, both the APC and the Th cell must "agree" that there is a problem before the Th cell can be activated. By requiring that Th cells only recognize presented antigen, Mother Nature guarantees that the decision to activate the deadly adaptive immune system is made by a committee, not by a single Th cell. In addition, because class II molecules present small fragments of proteins, the number of targets that a Th cell can "see" far exceeds those available for viewing in a large, folded protein -- just as with class I presentation.

ANTIGEN PRESENTING CELLS

Before a CTL can kill or a helper T cell can "help," both must be activated. To be activated, T cells must recognize their cognate antigen presented by an MHC molecule. But this is not enough. They must also receive a second, co-stimulatory signal. Only certain cells are equipped to provide this co-stimulation: the professional antigen presenting cells (APCs). Co-stimulation usually involves a protein on the surface of the antigen presenting cell called B7 that "plugs into" a protein called CD28 on the surface of the T cell.

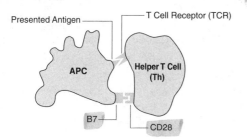

So far, three types of cells have been identified that can function as professional antigen presenting cells: macrophages, dendritic cells, and activated B cells. It's interesting to note that all of these professional APCs are white blood cells that start life in the bone marrow, and then migrate out to various sites in the body. Since new blood cells are made continuously, APCs can be replenished as needed.

MACROPHAGES

You recall that macrophages are sentinel cells that stand guard over those areas of your body that are exposed to the outside world. These are very adaptable cells that can function as garbage collectors, antigen presenting cells, or ferocious killers, depending on the signals they receive from the microenvironment in which they reside. In a resting state, macrophages are good at tidying up, but they are not much good as antigen presenting cells. The reason is that unless they are activated, macrophages don't express adequate levels of MHC or co-stimulatory molecules. Only when macrophages are activated by battle cytokines such as IFN-γ is the expression of MHC and co-stimulatory molecules upregulated so that macrophages can function as APCs. This system of activation before presentation makes great sense: Macrophages efficiently present antigen only when there has been an invasion, and there is something dangerous in the area to present.

DENDRITIC CELLS

The second professional antigen presenting cell is the dendritic cell (DC). The story about dendritic cells is quite interesting, because until just a few years ago, these cells were considered to be only a curiosity. The first DCs described were "Langerhans" cells that are found in the skin, but it is now recognized that DCs are found in the layer of cells that protects all exposed surfaces (the "epithelial" layer). In fact, this once obscure cell is now thought to be the most important of all the antigen presenting cells, because it can efficiently activate virgin T cells.

Dendritic cells have a characteristic starfish shape, and in a resting state, they express some B7 and relatively low levels of MHC molecules on their surfaces. But there's a subtlety here. Although resting DCs don't have many MHC molecules on their surfaces, they do have large internal stores of class II MHC molecules that are just waiting to be loaded. And the way these "reserve" MHC molecules are loaded for presentation to Th cells is really sweet. Here's how it works:

In normal tissues, DCs are wildly phagocytic -- they take up about four times their volume of extracellular fluid per hour. Mostly, they just drink it in and spit it back out. However, if an invader enters that tissue and it becomes a battle site, the lifestyle of the dendritic cell changes dramatically. When TNF, secreted by battling macrophages, binds to receptors on the surface of the dendritic cell, phagocytosis ceases, and the DC leaves the tissues and migrates through the lymphatic system to the nearest lymph node. When it arrives there, those antigens that were picked up at the battle scene are loaded onto the "reserve" MHC II molecules and displayed, so that surface expression of MHC II is dramatically increased. During its journey, the DC also upregulates expression of B7 co-stimulatory molecules, so that when it reaches the lymph node, the dendritic cell has everything it needs to activate virgin Th cells -- high levels of MHC II and high levels of B7.

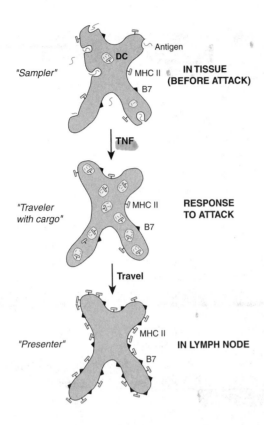

Now, why do you think it would be a good idea to have DCs that are wildly phagocytic in the tissues cease phagocytosis when they begin their journey to the lymph node? Exactly! Dendritic cells take a "snapshot" of what is happening on the "front lines," carry this image to the lymph node, and activate virgin T cells whose T cell receptors recognize the invader. You remember that lymph nodes are "dating bars" where T cells hang out, waiting to be activated. So the traveling dendritic cells actually bring the antigen from the battle to where the T cells are located. And why would you want battle cytokines such as TNF to trigger the migration of DCs to the lymph node? Of course! You want DCs to travel and present antigen only if a battle is on. Can you imagine a better system for antigen presentation? I don't think so!

T cells must be continuously re-stimulated, otherwise they think the battle has been won, and they go back to a resting state or die of neglect. Out in the tissues, the relatively low levels of MHC and B7 expression on DCs is sufficient to re-stimulate T cells that have already been activated, and which have traveled out into the tissues to join the battle. So dendritic cells can function to activate virgin T cells in lymph nodes and to re-stimulate experienced T cells at the battle scene.

ACTIVATED B CELLS

The third professional APC is the activated B cell. A virgin B cell is not much good at antigen presentation, because it expresses only low levels of MHC II and little or no B7. However, once a B cell has been activated, the levels of MHC II and B7 on its surface increase dramatically. As a result, an experienced B cell is able to act as an antigen presenting cell for Th cells. The current thinking is that B cells are not used as APCs during the initial stages of an infection, because at that time they are still naive -- they haven't been activated. However, later in the course of the infection or during subsequent infections, presentation of antigen by experienced B cells is thought to play an important role. Indeed, B cells have one great advantage over the other APCs -- B cells can concentrate antigen for presentation. Here's how this works:

When the B cell receptor binds to its cognate antigen, the whole complex of BCR and antigen is removed from the surface and taken into the cell. Once inside the cell, the antigen is processed, bound to MHC II molecules, and transported to the cell surface for presentation.

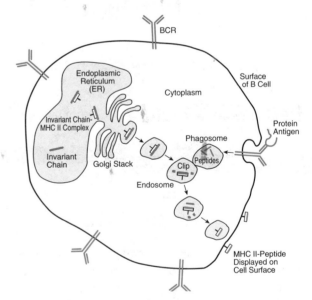

Because BCRs have a high affinity for antigen, the B cell acts like a magnet, collecting antigen for presentation to Th cells. Because a minimum number of T cell receptors must bind to antigen for a Th cell to be activated, it is estimated that B cells have a 100- to 10,000-fold advantage over other APCs in presenting antigen when there is relatively little of it around. So the first time an invader is encountered, the B cells are all virgins, and the important APCs are dendritic cells and macrophages. If this same invader is encountered again, however, the experienced, memory B cells become very important APCs, because they can get the adaptive immune response cranked up quickly by concentrating small amounts of antigen for presentation.

Now that you understand how antigens are presented and why presentation by class I and II MHC molecules is such a great idea, we need to turn our attention to the cells that are "looking at" these two kinds of display -- the helper T cell and the CTL. How these cells react to presented antigen is the subject of our next lecture.

SUMMARY FIGURE

You will notice that our summary figure now includes antigen presenting cells with their MHC and B7 molecules.

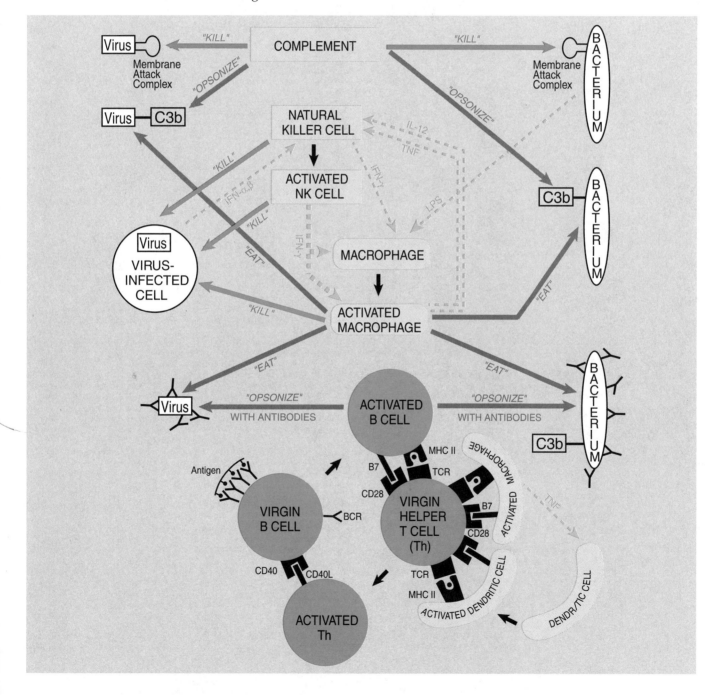

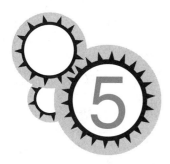

T CELLS AND CYTOKINES

REVIEW

In the last lecture we talked about MHC molecules and antigen presenting cells. You remember that there are two kinds of MHC molecules: class I and class II. Both molecules function as billboards that display either what is going on inside the cell (class I) or outside the cell (class II). For example, when a virus infects a cell, it takes over the cellular biosynthetic machinery, and uses it to produce proteins encoded by the virus. Some of these proteins are cut up into small pieces (peptides) by the proteasome, and carried by the TAP transporters into the endoplasmic reticulum (ER). There the peptides are "interviewed" by class I molecules. Those that are about nine amino acids in length with appropriate amino acids at their ends are bound in the grooves of class I MHC molecules, and transported to the surface of the cell. By scanning the MHC I-peptide complexes displayed there, cytotoxic lymphocytes (CTLs) can "look into a cell" to determine whether it has been infected and should be killed. This type of display, in which viral proteins are cut up into small pieces, has several advantages over a display of intact viral proteins. First, most viral proteins are normally not transported to the cell surface, so these proteins would never be seen by CTLs. Further, because protein folding can hide large portions of a protein from view, chopping a protein up into small peptides reveals many potential CTL targets that would be inaccessible in an intact protein. All in all, MHC class I display is a wonderful idea, because it greatly increases the probability that CTLs will recognize an infected cell.

Class II MHC molecules are billboards designed to alert helper T cells that a battle is being waged. For example, virus particles or viral debris can be taken up by antigen presenting cells, and presented to Th cells by class II MHC molecules. Class II molecules are assembled in the ER, just like class I molecules, but because invariant chain proteins occupy their binding grooves, class II molecules do not pick up peptides in the ER. Instead, the class II-invariant chain complex is transported out of the ER and into another cellular compartment called an endosome. There they meet up with proteins that have been taken into the cell by phagocytosis and cut up into peptides by enzymes. These peptides then replace the invariant chains that have been guarding the grooves of the class II molecules, and the MHC-peptide complexes are transported to the cell surface for display to Th cells. By this clever mechanism, class II molecules avoid peptides derived from proteins made in the cell, and pick up peptides derived from proteins taken in from outside the cell.

In addition to expressing class I and class II molecules, an antigen presenting cell must also provide the co-stimulatory signals required for T cell activation. Although activated macrophages and B cells have the "right stuff" to function as APCs for experienced T cells, it is likely that the most important APC for virgin T cells is the dendritic cell. This amazing cell picks up antigen out in the tissues, and under the influence of cytokines generated by other cells engaged in battle, migrates with its cargo of "battle antigen" to the nearest lymph node. There, the dendritic cell upregulates expression of MHC II and co-stimulatory molecules, and displays the peptides that it has collected out in the tissues. Thus, the dendritic cell effectively takes a snapshot of what is going on in the battle zone, carries it to the place where T cells are plentiful, and does its "show and tell" thing to activate Th cells.

T CELLS

In this lecture, we're going to focus on T cells -- how they are activated, and what they do. To begin, let's talk about T cell receptors (TCRs) -- those molecules on the surface of the T cell that function as the cell's windows on the world. Without these receptors, T cells would be flying blind with no way to sense what's going on outside.

T CELL RECEPTORS

TCRs come in two flavors: αβ and γδ. Each type of receptor is composed of two proteins, either α and β or γ and δ . Like the heavy and light chains of the B cell receptor, the genes for α β, γ, and δ are assembled by mixing and matching gene segments. As a result of a high stakes "card game" between chromosomes, each T cell ends up with either an αβ or a γδ receptor, but not both. Moreover, all the TCRs on a given T cell generally are identical, although there are exceptions to this rule.

Over 95% of the T cells in circulation have αβ T cell receptors and express either a CD4 or CD8 "co-receptor" molecule in addition to the αβ proteins. In contrast, most γδ T cells do not express either CD4 or CD8. T cells with γδ receptors are most abundant in areas like the intestine, the uterus, and the tongue which are in contact with the outside world. Interestingly, mice have lots of γδ T cells in the epidermal layer of their skin, but humans do not. This serves to remind us that so far as the immune system is concerned, humans are not just big mice.

Although αβ TCRs are thought to be about as diverse as BCRs, γδ receptors are less diverse. For example, the receptors of γδ T cells in the tongue and uterus tend to favor certain gene segments during rearrangement, whereas γδ receptors in the intestine prefer other sets of gene segments. The thinking here is that, like players on the innate immune system team, γδ T cells stand watch on the "front lines," and have receptors that are "tuned" to recognize invaders that commonly enter at certain locations.

Much about γδ T cells is still mysterious. For example, it is not known where these cells are educated. T cells with αβ receptors are taught in the thymus not to react to our own self peptides. Although γδ T cells are also found in the thymus, nude mice that lack a functional thymus still have functional γδ T cells. It is also not known exactly what it is that γδ T cells recognize. They may recognize antigen presented by "non-classical" MHC molecules that are different from the class I and class II MHC molecules we have talked about. There is also evidence that some γδ T cells recognize unpresented antigen in the same way that B cells do. Finally, the exact function of these cells is not clear, although there is speculation that γδ T cells recognize and kill cells that get "stressed" when they are infected with intracellular parasites.

Much more is known about T cells with αβ receptors. These receptors recognize a complex between a peptide and an MHC molecule on the surface of a cell. What I mean by "MHC-peptide complex" is a peptide bound in the groove of an MHC molecule. I use the word "complex" to emphasize the fact that the TCR recognizes both the peptide and the MHC molecule. A given T cell will have receptors that recognize either peptides associated with class I MHC molecules or with class II MHC molecules, but not both. Recognition by the TCR of an MHC-peptide complex takes place in several stages. First, adhesion molecules on the surface of the APC bind to their adhesion partners on the T cell, and bring the two cells together. This interaction is nonspecific and not very strong, but it gives the TCRs a chance to scan the MHC-peptide complexes on the surface of the APC to see if there is a match. If the TCRs do not see their cognate antigen on the APC billboard, the cells part, and the T cell goes on to scan other APCs.

If, however, the TCRs do find their match, the co-receptor molecules (either CD4 or CD8) on the surface of the T cell bind to the MHC molecules on the APC and strengthen the interaction between the two cells. Specifically, T cells with CD8 co- receptors (CD8$^+$ T cells) almost always interact with class I MHC molecules, and CD4$^+$ T cells almost always bind to class II MHC. Once the CD4 or CD8 molecules have engaged the appropriate MHC molecule, more adhesion molecules localize to the region of contact between the two cells, and the bond between the APC and the T cell strengthens. So the sequence of early events in T cell activation is: non-specific adhesion, TCR recognition of MHC-peptide, and stronger cell-cell adhesion.

HOW T CELL RECEPTORS SIGNAL

Once the TCR has recognized its cognate antigen presented by the MHC molecule, the next step is to transmit a signal from the surface of the cell, where recognition takes place, to the nucleus of the cell. The idea is that for the T cell to switch from a resting state to a state of activation, gene expression must be altered, and these genes are, of course, located in the cell's nucleus. Normally, this type of signaling across the cell membrane involves a transmembrane protein that has two parts: an external region whose job is to bind to a molecule that is outside the cell (called a ligand), and an internal region that initiates a biochemical cascade which conveys the "ligand bound" signal to the nucleus. Here the TCR runs into a bit of a problem. As is true of the BCR, the αβ TCR has a perfectly fine extracellular domain that can bind to its ligand (the combination of MHC molecule and peptide), but the cytoplasmic tails of these proteins are only about three amino acids long -- too short to do any signaling.

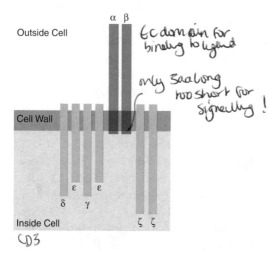

(handwritten annotations:) EC domain for binding to ligand

only 3aa long too short for signalling !

CD3

To handle the signaling part, Mother Nature had to add a few bells and whistles to the TCR: a complex of proteins collectively called CD3. In humans, this signaling complex is made up of four different proteins: γ, δ, ε, and ζ (gamma, delta, epsilon, and zeta). Please note, however, that the γ and δ proteins that are part of the CD3 complex are <u>not</u> the same as the γ and δ proteins that make up the γδ T cell receptor. The CD3 proteins are anchored in the cell membrane, and have cytoplasmic tails that are long enough to signal just fine. As with the BCR, signaling by the TCR involves clustering TCRs together in one area of the T cell surface, so that a threshold number of kinase enzymes is recruited by the cytoplasmic tails of the CD3 proteins to start the activation signal on its way to the nucleus.

Although the details about how this signaling works are still pretty sketchy, there are some interesting points about this six-protein, T cell receptor. First, the whole complex of proteins (α, β, γ, δ, ε, ζ) is transported to the cell surface as a unit. If any one of these proteins fails to be made, you don't get a TCR on the surface. So most immunologists consider the functional, mature TCR to be this whole complex of proteins. After all, the α and β proteins are great for recognition, but they can't signal. And the γ, δ, ε, and ζ proteins signal just fine, but they are totally blind to what's going on outside the cell. You need both parts to make it work.

Back when the α and β chains of the TCR were first discovered, it was thought that the TCR was just an on/off switch whose function was only to signal activation. But now that you have heard about the four CD3 proteins, let me ask you: Does this look like a simple on/off switch? No way. Mother Nature certainly wouldn't make an on/off switch with six proteins. No, this TCR is quite versatile -- it can send signals that result in very different outcomes, depending on how, when, and where it is triggered. For example, during their education in the thymus, T cell receptors are used to trigger suicide (death by apoptosis) if the TCR recognizes MHC plus self peptides. Later, if the TCR recognizes its cognate antigen presented by MHC, but the T cell does not receive the required co-stimulatory signals, that T cell is neutered (anergized) so it can't function. And, of course, when a TCR is engaged by cognate antigen and co-stimulatory signals are available, the TCR signals activation. So this same T cell receptor, depending on the situation, signals death, anergy, or activation. In fact, there are now documented cases in which the change of a single amino acid in a presented peptide can change the signal from activation to death! Clearly this is no on/off switch, and immunologists are working very hard to understand exactly how TCR signaling is "wired" and what factors (e.g., co-stimulation) influence the signaling outcome.

CO-STIMULATION

In addition to having their T cell receptors ligated by MHC-peptide, T cells must also receive co-stimulatory signals before they can be activated. During activation, a threshold number of TCRs must be engaged before there will be enough enzymatic activity generated to dispatch the "receptor engaged" signal to the nucleus. Measurements suggest that <u>without</u> co-stimulation, a huge number of TCRs on a virgin T cell would have to bind MHC-peptide complexes on the APC before signaling would occur -- so many in fact that this probably never would happen. In contrast, if the T cell receives appropriate co-stimulation, the number of TCRs that must be bound (ligated) is reduced dramatically. Thus, one effect of receiving the second, co-stimulatory signal is to lower the threshold number of TCRs that must be engaged by MHC-peptide.

The best studied co-stimulation involves a molecule expressed on the surface of antigen presenting cells called B7. A second, closely related molecule has now been discovered, so immunologists are calling these B7-1 and B7-2. B7 molecules provide co-stimulation to T cells by plugging into receptors on the T cell surface. So far, two of these receptors have been identified: CD28 and CTLA-4. Most T cells express CD28. In contrast, CTLA-4 is only expressed after a T cell has been activated. Current thinking is that B7 proteins on APCs ligate the CD28 receptor on virgin T cells, and provide the co-stimulatory signal necessary for activation. Then, once the cell has been activated, ligation of CTLA-4 by B7 helps to eventually turn off or "deactivate" the T cell. It's very important, of course, that the immune response be turned off, once its job is done. Otherwise, we'd fill up with activated B and T cells that could protect us against enemies from our past, but not against present or future invaders. Using CTLA-4 ligation as a negative regulator of T cell activation seems to be one way this is accomplished.

In addition to surface molecules like B7, cytokines secreted by APCs also contribute to co-stimulation. What is now being appreciated is that different antigen presenting cells in different locations express different mixtures of co-stimulatory molecules and cytokines. For example, macrophages express B7-1 and the cytokine, IL-l; dendritic cells express roughly equal amounts of B7-1 and B7-2; and activated B cells express more B7-1 than B7-2. So the emerging picture is that different APCs provide different kinds of co-stimulatory signals to T cells, and these different signals can influence the types of cytokines that Th cells secrete.

There is a final, important point about co-stimulation. In their resting state, antigen presenting cells like macrophages, dendritic cells, and B cells do not express enough of the B7 co-stimulator on their sur-

faces to activate naive T cells. So APCs must be "activated" before they can present antigen effectively. What is interesting about this is that the signals which activate APCs (e.g., TNF and IFN-γ) come either directly or indirectly from the innate immune system. As a result, it is the innate immune system's reaction to danger that makes it possible to activate the adaptive immune system. In a real sense, the innate system "gives permission" for the adaptive system to be activated by controlling the expression of co-stimulatory molecules on APCs.

CD4 AND CD8 CO-RECEPTORS

Doesn't it seem that Mother Nature got carried away with the CD4 and CD8 co-receptors? I mean, there are two proteins, α and β, to use for antigen recognition; and four more, γ, δ, ϵ, and ζ, to use for signaling. Wouldn't you think that would do it? Apparently not, so there must be essential features of the system that require CD4 and CD8 co-receptors. Let's see what these might be.

Killer T cells and helper T cells perform two very different functions, and they "look at" two different molecules, class I or class II MHC, to get their cues. But how do CTLs know to focus on peptides presented by class I molecules on virus-infected cells, and how do Th cells know to scan APCs for peptides presented by class II? After all, it wouldn't be so great if a CTL got confused, recognized a class II-peptide complex on an APC, and killed that cell. So here's where CD4 and CD8 come in. CTLs generally express CD8 and Th cells usually express CD4, and these co-receptor molecules are designed to clip onto either class I MHC (CD8) or class II MHC molecules (CD4), and strengthen the adhesion between the T cell and the APC.

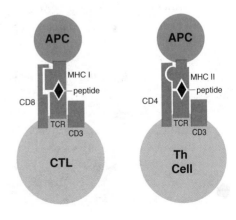

So CD4 and CD8 co-receptors function to focus the attention of CTLs and Th cells on the proper MHC molecule. But there is more to the story, because it turns out that CD4 and CD8 are signaling molecules just like the CD3 complex of proteins. Both CD4 and CD8 have tails that extend through the cell wall and into the interior (cytoplasm) of the cell, and both of these tails have the right characteristics to signal. In addition, because CD4 is a single protein and CD8 is composed of two different proteins, the signals that these co-receptors send are likely to be quite different -- perhaps as different as "help" and "kill." In contrast to the CD3 molecules, which are glued rather tightly to the αβ T cell receptor on the cell surface, the CD4 and CD8 co-receptors usually are only loosely associated with the TCR/CD3 proteins. The latest thinking is that the MHC molecule on the APC actually functions as a "clamp" that brings together the TCR/CD3 complex and the CD4 or CD8 molecule on the surface of the T cell, and that this clustering of TCR/CD3 with CD4 or CD8 greatly amplifies the signal sent by the TCR.

When T cells begin maturing in the thymus, they express both co-receptors on their surfaces. Immunologists call them CD4$^+$CD8$^+$ cells. Then, as they mature, expression of one or the other of these co-receptors is downregulated, and a cell becomes either CD4$^+$ or CD8$^+$. So how does a given T cell decide whether it will express CD4 or CD8 when it grows up? Well, immunologists are not any more certain about how T cells decide to be CD4$^+$ or CD8$^+$ than they are about how B cells decide to be plasma cells or memory cells. Some think that it is just a random process in which T cells downregulate expression of one type of co-receptor. Others propose that if a TCR happens to bind, say, to a class I molecule on the surface of a cell in the thymus, the CD8 molecule "clips on" and a signal is sent to downregulate CD4 expression. Unfortunately, there are experimental results that argue for each of these models, so the question of how T cells decide on their co-receptor molecule is still unanswered.

EVENTS DURING T CELL ACTIVATION

I'll bet your picture of T cell activation is that antigen presenting cells flit from T cell to T cell, activating them. This certainly used to be how I visualized the process. As it turns out, however, activation of a T cell takes quite some time -- generally from eight to twenty-four hours -- so "flitting" is not exactly what these cells do. During these hours, several interesting things happen. Early in activation, expression of surface adhesion molecules is upregulated, so that the "glue" holding the APC and T cell together strengthens. This is important for keeping these cells together for the activation period, because the binding between the T cell receptor and the MHC-peptide complex is rather weak. In fact, the ability to express the adhesion molecules required to keep APCs and T cells together is one feature that sets APCs apart from "ordinary" cells.

Also during activation, growth factor receptors appear on the surface of the T cell (e.g., receptors for IL-2). This makes sense, because after T cells are activated, they must proliferate (clonal selection, right?), and this proliferation is driven by cytokines like IL-2 that act as growth factors. Resting T cells don't express receptors for these growth factors -- that's why they are "resting."

CYTOKINES SECRETED BY Th CELLS

When virgin T cells are first activated, the major cytokine they secrete is IL-2. Since activated T cells also have receptors for IL-2, what we have is a case of "self stimulation" (autocrine stimulation) in which a T cell both produces and reacts to its own growth factor. As a result of this autocrine stimulation, recently-activated T cells proliferate to increase the number of T cells specific for the invader. After all, a single T cell isn't going to be much help against a raging infection. Once Th cells have proliferated to build up a clone, they may be re-stimulated by an APC, and if they are, they begin to secrete other cytokines such as IFN-γ, IL-4, IL-5, IL-10, and TNF. Generally, a single Th cell doesn't secrete all these different cytokines. In fact, Th cells tend to secrete subsets of all the possible cytokines. These subsets are frequently of two general types: a "Th1" subset that includes IL-2, IFN-γ, and TNF; and a "Th2" subset that includes interleukins 4, 5, and 10.

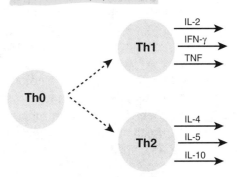

You shouldn't take this to mean, however, that there are only two subsets of cytokines that can be secreted by Th cells. In fact, immunologists initially had a hard time finding helper cells that secreted the Th1 or Th2 cytokine subsets in humans. So while it is clear that there are Th cells which secrete mixtures of cytokines that don't conform to the Th1/Th2 paradigm, the concept of Th1 and Th2 subsets turns out to be quite useful in trying to make sense of the mixture of cytokines (the cytokine "profile") that Th cells secrete.

Why do you think it makes sense that different Th cells secrete different subsets of the possible cytokines? Let's review the functions of the cytokines that make up the Th1 and Th2 subsets, and I think you'll see what Mother Nature is up to. The "classical" Th1 cytokines are IFN-γ, IL-2, and TNF. IFN-γ is a cytokine that primes macrophages, and influences B cells during class switching to produce IgG3 antibodies that are good at opsonizing viruses and bacteria and at fixing complement. TNF activates primed macrophages and NK cells. IL-2 is a growth factor that stimulates CTLs and NK cells to proliferate. So the Th1 cytokines are the perfect package to help defend against a viral or bacterial attack, because they instruct the innate and adaptive systems to produce cells and antibodies that are effective against bacteria and viruses.

Now let's look at the Th2 profile of cytokines. IL-4 is a growth factor for B cells that can also influence B cells to class switch to produce IgE antibodies. IL-5 is also a growth factor for B cells, and it can influence B cells to produce IgA antibodies. So the Th2 cytokine profile is just the ticket if you need to make lots of antibodies to defend against a parasitic (IgE) or mucosal (IgA) infection.

What's happening here is really neat. By secreting the appropriate set of cytokines, Th cells can help produce an immune response that is appropriate to a given invader -- so that the punishment fits the crime. The Th cell is the quarterback of the immune system, and this is how the plays are called -- by secreting these hormone-like cytokines that direct the immune response.

The next logical question, then, is: How are the Th cytokine profiles determined? Here the picture gets a little fuzzy, but I'll tell you the latest thinking. When Th cells are first activated, they make the growth factor IL-2, which causes them to go through rounds of proliferation to build up their numbers. Then, when Th cells are re-stimulated, they begin to produce other cytokines, so it is at the re-stimulation stage that the cytokine profile is usually determined. The initial decision on which cytokines Th cells will produce is driven by the co-stimulatory molecules provided by the APCs that do the re-stimulating, and by the mixture of cytokines in the microenvironment in which the re-stimulation takes place. For example, macrophages responding to a viral or bacterial attack secrete IL-12. This cytokine influences Th cells to produce Th1 cytokines -- the cytokine profile that will help the innate and adaptive systems defend against viruses and bacteria.

In contrast, if Th cells are re-activated in an environment in which there is a lot of IL-4 (which is usually the case during a parasitic attack), they are influenced to secrete cytokines of the Th2 subset -- cytokines that are perfect for defending against parasites. The bottom line is that the environment in which Th cells are re-stimulated influences uncommitted Th cells to secrete a Th1 or Th2 profile of cytokines.

The second influence on the cytokine profile secreted by a Th cell is positive or negative feedback from other Th cells in the neighborhood. Here's how this works. Th1 cells secrete IFN-γ, which, together with danger signals like the bacterial molecule LPS, helps activate macrophages. When macrophages are activated, they secrete IL-12, which is the major cytokine that influences Th cells to secrete the Th1 profile of cytokines. So a positive feedback loop is set up in which the cytokines produced by committed Th1 cells influence the decision of undecided (Th0) helper T cells to join the Th1 club.

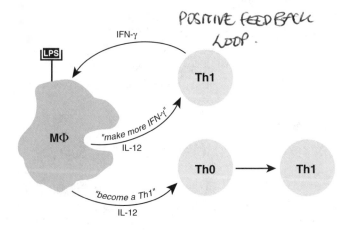

The same sort of thing goes on with Th cells that are of the Th2 type, because these cells secrete IL-4 -- the major cytokine that influences Th0 cells to secrete the Th2 profile. So in both cases, cytokines secreted by committed Th cells either directly or indirectly recruit other, uncommitted Th cells to secrete the same mixture of cytokines.

Once a Th cell has made a choice, it begins to secrete its own growth factor: Th1 cells secrete IL-2 which is a growth factor that drives Th1 cell proliferation; and Th2 cells secrete their favorite growth factor, IL-4, that causes them to proliferate.

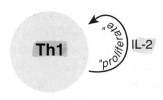

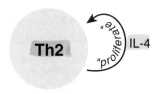

So not only do the cytokines secreted by each subset encourage new Th cells to fall into step, but these cytokines also cause the selected Th cells to proliferate to build up their numbers.

Finally, there is also <u>negative</u> feedback at work. IFN-γ made by Th1 cells actually decreases the rate of proliferation of Th2 cells, so that fewer Th2 cells will be produced.

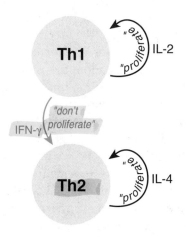

On the other side of the picture, one of the Th2 cytokines, IL-10, acts to decrease the rate of proliferation of Th1 cells.

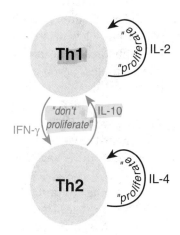

In addition, IL-4 (in humans) downregulates expression of IL-12 and TNF by activated macrophages, breaking the macrophage-Th1 positive feedback loop.

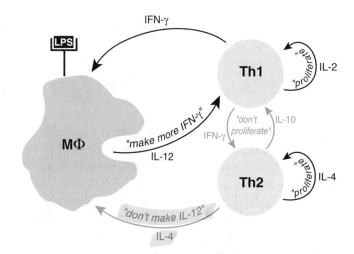

In mice, this negative-feedback function is performed by IL-10, not IL-4. Of course, it isn't the name of the cytokine that's important here. What's important is the <u>concept</u>: once a Th subset has been established, positive and negative feedback tend to "lock in" this particular subset. In addition, growth factors secreted by the "selected" Th subset cause cells of this subset to proliferate and "outgrow" cells of the other subset.

Now there is one very important point here that I want to make sure you understand. When we talk about influencing the immune response toward a Th1 or Th2 cytokine profile, we are talking about something very local. That's why I used the term, "microenvironment." Clearly, you wouldn't want every Th cell in your body to be of the Th1 type, because then you'd have no way to defend against a respiratory infection. Conversely, you wouldn't want to have all Th2 cells, because the IgA antibodies made in response to the Th2 cytokines would be useless if you get a bacterial infection in your big toe. So if you were designing this system, you would fix it so that the local environment biased Th cells to secrete the cytokines that would defend you best against invaders commonly encountered in that neighborhood -- and that's exactly what happens!

There is one other important point about the establishment of helper T cell subsets. Because the innate system is activated earlier in an infection than is the adaptive system, the innate system usually establishes the cytokine environment that determines the initial commitment of Th cells to secrete either a Th1 or Th2 profile of cytokines. Thus, the innate immune system not only informs the adaptive system when there is danger, but it also plays a large part in determining what weapons the adaptive system will make.

AN EXAMPLE OF WHAT HELPER T CELLS DO

We have already talked quite a bit about Th cells and how they direct the immune response by secreting cytokines, but there is one example of this I think you'll find interesting. It's called delayed type hypersensitivity (DTH), and it was first observed by Robert Koch when he was doing his famous studies on tuberculosis back in the latter part of the nineteenth century. Koch purified a protein, tuberculin, from the bacterium that causes tuberculosis, and he used this protein to devise the famous "tuberculin skin test." If you've had this test, you'll recall that a nurse injected tuberculin under your skin, and told you to check that area in a few days. If you had not been exposed to the tuberculosis bacterium, you saw little or no reaction. In contrast, if you had been infected with TB, the site of injection became red and swollen. This reaction is an example of delayed type hypersensitivity, and here's what's happening:

When you are injected, dendritic cells in your skin (the so-called "Langerhans" cells) take up the tuberculin and use class II MHC molecules to display fragments of the tuberculin protein. If you have active TB or have been infected with it in the past, your immune system will already include experienced Th cells that can recognize the tuberculin fragments displayed by the dendritic cells, and be re-activated. You remember that dendritic cells in the tissues express enough MHC and B7 molecules to re-stimulate experienced T cells, but not enough of these molecules to activate naive T cells.

Now the fun begins, because when these Th cells are re-activated, they will secrete IFN-γ and TNF. These Th1-type cytokines will activate resident tissue macrophages near the site of injection, and will help recruit neutrophils and additional macrophages to the area. The result will be a local inflammatory reaction, with the usual redness and swelling that we talked about in the first lecture. What is interesting here is that delayed type hypersensitivity is both specific and non-specific. The specificity comes from Th cells that direct the immune response after specifically recognizing the tuberculin peptide presented by dendritic cells. The non-specific part of the reaction includes neutrophils and macrophages that are recruited and activated by cytokines secreted by the Th cells. This is yet another example of the cooperation that goes on between adaptive and innate immune systems. The reaction to tuberculin is delayed for a couple days, because circulating Th cells must be re-activated, proliferate, and secrete cytokines; and neutrophils and additional macrophages must be recruited from the blood.

You may be wondering why the tuberculin used for the test doesn't activate naive T cells, so that the next time you are tested, you get a positive reaction. The reason is that the tuberculin protein does not, by itself, cause an inflammatory reaction, and you remember that dendritic cells only leave the epithelium and travel to a lymph node if they receive battle cytokines like TNF. So if a protein is injected under the skin and does not cause inflammation, the dendritic cells don't travel, and the adaptive immune system doesn't get activated. Of course, if the tuberculin were injected at the site in your big toe where a battle was already raging against the bacteria from that now-famous splinter, then the tuberculin might be carried by dendritic cells to a lymph node where tuberculin-specific, virgin T cells could be activated. This illustrates again how important the innate immune system is for initiating an immune response: If your innate system does not recognize an invader as dangerous and put up a fight, your adaptive system will usually just ignore the invader.

WHAT KILLER T CELLS DO

In contrast to helper T cells, which are cytokine factories, cytotoxic lymphocytes (CTLs) are, as the name implies, lymphocytes that kill. This killing, however, is also directed by Th cells, because most CTLs depend on the growth factor IL-2 to proliferate, and Th1 cells are major suppliers of this cytokine. Therefore, in order to mount a strong CTL response to a viral infection, it is important that helper T cells are biased towards secreting a Th1 cytokine profile, so there will be plenty of IL-2 around.

Killing by CTLs -- for example, killing of virus-infected cells -- requires cell-cell contact, and CTLs actually have several weapons they can use. The first involves the production of the protein, perforin, that can open a hole in the target cell. Perforin is a close relative of the C9 complement protein that is part of the membrane attack complex. Sometimes the holes made by perforin become so large and numerous that the cell dies, because the protected environment inside the cell is exposed to the outside world. This type of cell death is called necrosis. In other situations, CTLs kill by delivering an enzyme called granzyme B into the target cell. This enzyme is stored in little pouches inside the CTL. Once the CTL establishes contact with its target, granzyme B is dumped onto the target cell where it binds to receptor proteins and is taken inside. Once inside the target cell, granzyme B can trigger the cell to commit suicide. This kind of cell death is called apoptosis, and it usually involves destruction of the target cell's DNA by the target cell's own enzymes.

CTLs also can kill by using a protein on their surfaces called Fas ligand (FasL) that can bind to (ligate) the Fas protein on the surface of the target cell. When this happens, a suicide program is set in motion, and the cells die by apoptosis.

So CTLs have several different ways of killing their target cells, and the result is death either by necrosis or apoptosis. Although the end result is the same (a dead target cell), death by necrosis or apoptosis is quite different. In necrosis, enzymes and chemicals that usually are contained within the dying cell are released into the surrounding tissues where they can do real damage. In contrast, death by apoptosis is much cleaner, because as the cell dies, the contents of the cell are enclosed in pouches (vesicles). These vesicles are phagocytosed and destroyed by nearby macrophages as part of their garbage collecting duty. As a result, the contents of the target cell don't get out into the tissues to cause damage.

Triggering cells to die by apoptosis is an especially good way for CTLs to kill virus-infected cells, because the DNA of unassembled viruses is usually destroyed along with the target cell's DNA. Moreover, assembled viruses inside the infected target cell are enclosed in vesicles and destroyed by macrophages, thereby preventing the viral infection from spreading.

EPILOGUE

As we come to the end of this lecture, you should now be familiar with all of the major players of the innate and adaptive immune systems. As I'm sure you now understand, these players form a "network" in which they work together to defend us from disease. For this network to function, however, the movements of the various players must be carefully orchestrated to enhance cooperation between players, and to make sure that the appropriate weapons are delivered to the locations where they are needed within the body. How this all is accomplished is the subject of our next lecture.

SUMMARY FIGURE

Here is our final summary figure, showing both the innate and adaptive systems--and the network they form. Can you identify all the players, and do you understand how they interact with each other?

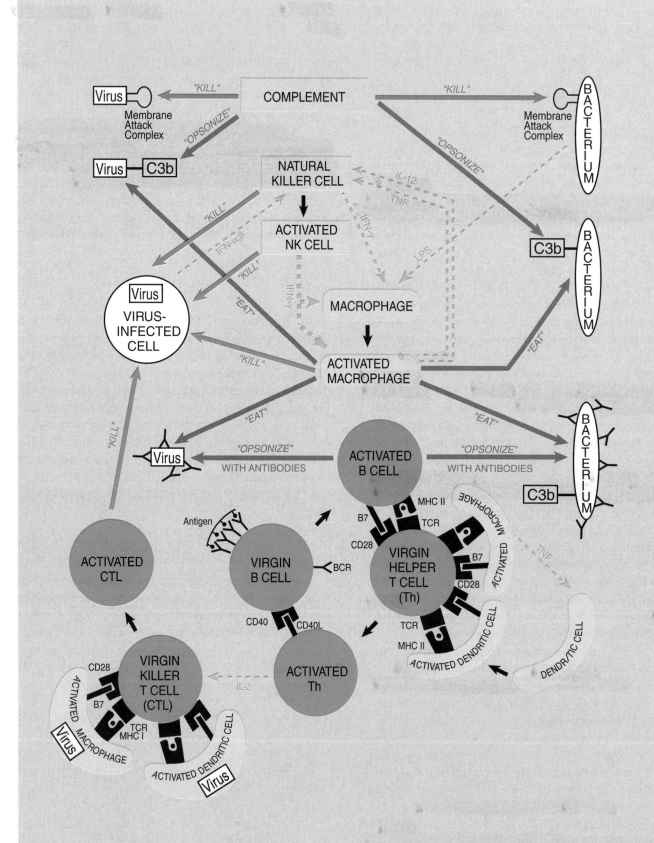

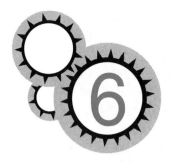

6

LYMPHOID ORGANS AND LYMPHOCYTE TRAFFICKING

REVIEW

In the last lecture, we talked about T cells and T cell activation, and as I'm sure you noticed, there are many similarities between T cells and B cells. As a way of reviewing what you've learned, let's discuss some of the ways that T and B cells are similar -- and different.

BCRs and TCRs both have "recognition" proteins that extend outside the cell, and which are made by a strategy of mixing and matching gene segments. For the BCR, these are the light and heavy chains that make up the antibody molecule. For the TCR, the molecules that recognize antigen are the α and β or γ and δ proteins. The recognition molecules of the TCR and the BCR have cytoplasmic tails that are too short to signal recognition, so additional molecules are required for this purpose. For the BCR, these signaling proteins are called Igα and Igβ, while for the TCR, signaling involves a complex of proteins called CD3.

In addition to recognition and signaling molecules, BCRs and TCRs also associate with co-receptor molecules that serve to amplify the signal that the receptor sends. For B cells this co-receptor is a surface protein (complement receptor) which recognizes antigen that has been opsonized by complement. If the BCR recognizes an antigen, and if that antigen is "decorated" with complement protein fragments, the antigen serves as a "clamp" that brings the BCR and the complement receptor together on the surface of the B cell, greatly amplifying the "receptor engaged" signal. As a result, B cells are much more easily activated (many fewer BCRs must be crosslinked) by antigen that has been opsonized by complement.

T cells also have co-receptors: Th cells express CD4 molecules on their surfaces, and CTLs express CD8 molecules. When a TCR binds to antigen presented by MHC I (CTL) or MHC II (Th cell), the co-receptor molecule on the T cell surface also binds to the MHC molecule. Thus, the MHC molecule functions as a "clamp" that brings together the TCR and the CD4 or CD8 co-receptor on the surface of the T cell. This serves to amplify the signal that is sent by the TCR to the nucleus, so that the T cell is much more easily activated (fewer TCRs must be crosslinked). Of course, this "clamping" only works for the "right" MHC type: MHC I for CTLs with CD8 co-receptors and MHC II for Th cells with CD4 co-receptors.

So co-receptors really are "focus" molecules. The B cell co-receptor helps B cells focus on antigens that have already been identified by the complement system as dangerous (those that have been opsonized). The CD4 co-receptor focuses the attention of Th cells on antigens displayed by class II MHC molecules, and the CD8 co-receptor focuses CTLs on antigens displayed by class I MHC molecules.

For B and T cells to be activated, their receptors must be clustered by antigen, because this crosslinking brings together many of their signaling molecules in a small region of the cell. When the density of signaling molecules is great enough, an enzymatic chain reaction is set off that conveys the "receptor engaged" signal to the cell's nucleus. While crosslinking of receptors is essential for activation, it is not enough. To be activated, naive B and T cells also require co-stimulatory signals which are not antigen specific. For B cell activation, a helper T cell can provide co-stimulation through a surface protein called CD40L that plugs into the CD40 protein on the B cell surface. For T cells, the main co-stimulation involves the CD28 protein on the surface of the T cell that is ligated by the B7 protein on an antigen presenting cell.

When B and T cells are activated, growth factor receptors appear on their surfaces. This allows them to proliferate in response to the appropriate growth factors, and to form a clone of cells that has the same antigen specificity. B and Th cells are also similar in that when they are re-stimulated, they get a chance to change the molecules they secrete. B cells can undergo class switching to produce IgG, IgA, or IgE antibodies in place of the default antibody class, IgM. The Th cell can secrete a whole list of cytokines in addition to, or instead of, the default cytokine, IL-2. In both cases, the change in isotype or cytokine profile is controlled by the cytokine environment of the B or Th cell.

In addition to these similarities, there are important differences between B cells and T cells. The BCR recognizes antigen in its "natural" state -- that is, antigen that has not been chopped up and bound to MHC molecules. This antigen can be a protein or almost any other organic molecule (e.g., a carbohydrate or a fat). In contrast, the αβ TCR only recognizes fragments of proteins that are presented by MHC molecules. So the BCR has much greater variety in the type of antigen it can recognize. However, because the TCR looks at small fragments of proteins, the TCR can recognize targets that might be hidden from view of the BCR when the protein is intact and folded up.

Of course, B and T cells have different functions. B cells secrete antibodies -- a non-membrane-anchored form of the BCR. In contrast, the TCR stays firmly anchored on the surface of the T cell. Experienced B cells can function as antigen presenting cells, but T cells cannot. CTLs can function as killers, but B cells do not kill. Finally, Th cells are major cytokine producers, whereas B cells usually produce cytokines only in small amounts.

During an infection, the rearranged heavy and light chain genes that make up B cell receptors can undergo somatic hypermutation and selection. As a result, the average affinity of the collection of BCRs increases. So in a sense, B cells can "draw from the deck" to try to get a better hand. In contrast, the TCR does not hypermutate, so T cells must be satisfied with the cards they are dealt. B cells are produced more or less continuously throughout the lifetime of a human, but most T cells are produced early in life. The reason is that the organ in which T cells mature, the thymus, steadily decreases in activity after puberty, so fewer and fewer freshly-minted T cells roll off the thymic assembly line as we get older. That's one reason why some viral diseases such as mumps, which are just a nuisance to a kid, can be deadly serious to an older person.

Certainly one of the most interesting parts of the last lecture was our discussion of how Mother Nature arranges to "let the punishment fit the crime." Because the immediate environment in which the Th cell is re-stimulated determines which cytokines it will produce, the Th cell is sensitive to what's going on around it. If it is re-stimulated in the midst of a bacterial or viral infection, a helper T cell tends to secrete a Th1 profile of cytokines that includes IFN-γ, TNF, and IL-2. These are especially appropriate for mounting a "cellular" defense against a viral or bacterial attack, because IL-2 encourages CTLs to proliferate, and IFN-γ and TNF help activate macrophages and NK cells. In contrast, if a Th cell is re-stimulated in the midst of a mucosal infection, it tends to secrete a Th2 cytokine profile that includes IL-4 and IL-5. These cytokines favor a strong antibody (sometimes called "humoral") defense. Because the innate system is activated earlier in an infection than is the adaptive system, the cytokine environment that determines the initial commitment of Th cells to secrete a Th1 or Th2 profile of cytokines is usually established by the innate system. Again we see the adaptive system following the innate system's lead.

SECONDARY LYMPHOID ORGANS AND LYMPHOCYTE TRAFFICKING

So far, we have talked about the various elements of the adaptive immune system without too much regard for where in the body things take place. In this lecture, I want to give you some spacial perspective by discussing the "geography" of the immune system.

When you think about it, the immune system's defense against an invader has three phases: recognition of danger, production of weapons specific for the invader, and transport of these weapons to the site of attack. Today we'll discuss when and where these three phases take place.

The recognition phase of the adaptive immune response takes place in the so-called "secondary lymphoid organs." These include the lymph nodes, the spleen, and the mucosal associated lymphoid tissue (called the MALT for short). You may be wondering: If these are the secondary lymphoid organs, what are the primary ones? The primary lymphoid organs are the places where B and T cells are born or receive their early training: the bone marrow and the thymus.

THE LYMPHOID FOLLICLE

All secondary lymphoid organs have one anatomical feature in common: they all contain lymphoid follicles. These follicles are critical for the functioning of the adaptive immune system, so we need to spend a little time getting familiar with them. Lymphoid follicles start life as "primary" lymphoid follicles: loose networks of follicular dendritic cells (FDCs) that are embedded in regions of the secondary lymphoid organs that are rich in B cells. So lymphoid follicles are really islands of follicular dendritic cells within a sea of B cells.

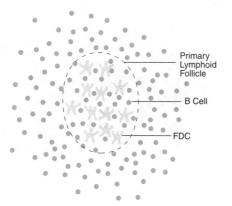

Primary Lymphoid Follicle

B Cell

FDC

Although FDCs have the classic starfish dendritic shape, they are very different from the dendritic cells (DCs) of the skin and mucosa that we have talked about before. Those dendritic cells, which function as professional antigen presenting cells, are white blood cells that are produced in the bone marrow, and which then migrate to their sentinel positions in tissues. In contrast, follicular dendritic cells are regular old cells (like skin cells or liver cells) that take up their final positions in the body as the embryo develops. In fact, follicular dendritic cells are already in place during the second trimester of gestation. Not only are the origins of follicular dendritic cells and antigen presenting dendritic cells quite different, these two types of starfish-shaped cells have very different functions. Whereas the role of dendritic APCs is to present antigen to T cells via MHC molecules, the function of follicular dendritic cells is to display antigen to B cells. Here's how this works:

Early in an infection, complement proteins bind to invaders, and some of this complement-opsonized antigen will be delivered by the lymph or blood to the secondary lymphoid organs. Follicular dendritic cells that reside in these organs have receptors on their surfaces that bind complement fragments, and as a result, follicular dendritic cells pick up and retain the opsonized antigen. In this way, follicular dendritic cells become "decorated" with antigens that are characteristic of the battle that is being waged out in the tissues. Later in infection, when antibodies have been produced, invaders opsonized by antibodies can also be captured by FDCs, because these cells have receptors that can bind to the constant regions of antibody molecules.

So the function of follicular dendritic cells is to capture opsonized antigen and to "advertize" this antigen to B cells. Those B cells that recognize their cognate antigens hanging from these follicular dendritic "trees" are retained for a while in the lymphoid follicle where they proliferate. Once this happens, the "follicle" begins to grow and to become the center of B cell development. Such an active lymphoid follicle is called a "secondary" lymphoid follicle or a "germinal center." The role of complement-opsonized antigen in triggering the development of a germinal center cannot be over emphasized: lymphoid follicles in humans who have a defective complement system never progress past the primary stage. This is another example of an important concept in immunology: For the adaptive immune system to respond, the innate system must first react to impending danger.

Once B cells have proliferated in germinal centers they become very "fragile." Unless they receive the proper "rescue" signals, they will commit suicide (die by apoptosis). Fortunately, helper T cells that have been activated in the T cell areas of the secondary lymphoid organs migrate to the lymphoid follicle. These activated Th cells express high levels of the CD40L protein that can plug into the CD40 protein on the surface of the B cell. When a B cell whose receptors are crosslinked receives this co-stimulatory signal, it is temporarily rescued from apoptotic death, and continues to proliferate. The rate at which these B cells multiply is truly amazing -- the number of B cells can double every six hours! These proliferating B cells push aside other B cells that have not been activated, and establish a region of the germinal center that is called the dark zone -- because it contains so many proliferating B cells that it looks dark under the microscope.

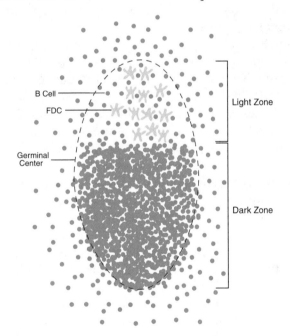

After a period of proliferation, some of the B cells will "decide" to become plasma B cells, while others will undergo somatic hypermutation to "fine tune" their receptors. After each round of mutation, the affinity of the mutated BCR is tested. Those B cells whose mutated BCRs do not have a high enough affinity for antigen to be efficiently crosslinked will die by apoptosis, and be eaten by macrophages in the germinal center. In contrast, B cells will be rescued from apoptosis if their receptors have a high enough affinity to be efficiently

crosslinked by antigen on FDCs, and if they receive co-stimulation from activated Th cells that are present in the light zone of the germinal center. The current picture is that B cells "cycle" between periods of proliferation in the dark zone and periods of testing in the light zone. Sometime during all this action, B cells can also switch the class of antibody they produce. This process is believed to take place in the light zone of the germinal center with the aid of activated Th cells.

In summary, lymphoid follicles are specialized regions of secondary lymphoid organs in which B cells percolate through a lattice of follicular dendritic cells that have captured opsonized antigen on their surfaces. B cells that encounter their cognate antigen and receive T cell help are rescued from death. These "saved" B cells proliferate and can undergo somatic hypermutation and isotype switching. Clearly lymphoid follicles are extremely important for B cell development. That's why all the secondary lymphoid organs have them.

HIGH ENDOTHELIAL VENULES

A second anatomical feature common to all secondary lymphoid organs except the spleen is the "high endothelial venule" (HEV). The reason the HEV is so important is that it is the "doorway" through which B and T cells enter these secondary lymphoid organs from the blood. Most endothelial cells that line the inside of blood vessels resemble overlapping shingles that are tightly "glued" to the cells adjacent to them to prevent the loss of blood cells into the tissues. In contrast, the blood vessels that collect blood from the capillary beds (the post-capillary venules) in most secondary lymphoid organs have endothelial cells that are shaped more like a column than like a shingle:

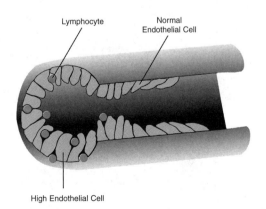

These tall cells are the high endothelial cells -- so a high endothelial venule is a special region in a blood vessel (venule) where there are high endothelial cells. Instead of being glued together, high endothelial cells are "spot welded." As a result, there is space between the cells of the HEV for lymphocytes to wriggle through. Actually, "wriggle" may not be quite the right term, because lymphocytes exit the blood very efficiently at these high endothelial venules: about 10,000 lymphocytes enter an average lymph node each second by passing between high endothelial cells!

A TOUR OF THE SECONDARY LYMPHOID ORGANS

Now that you are familiar with lymphoid follicles and high endothelial venules, we are ready to take a tour of some of the secondary lymphoid organs. On our tour today, we will visit a lymph node, a Peyer's patch (an example of the MALT), and the spleen. As we explore these organs, I want you to pay special attention to the "plumbing." How an organ is plumbed will give us clues about the purpose of the organ and how it functions.

LYMPH NODES

The lymph node is a plumber's dream. This organ has incoming lymphatics which bring lymph into the node, and outgoing lymphatics through which lymph exits the node. In addition, there are arterioles that bring blood into the lymph node, and veins through which blood exits. If you look carefully at this figure, you can also see the high endothelial venules.

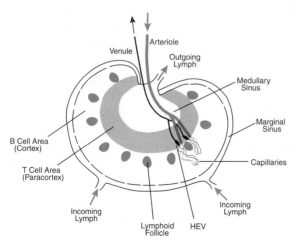

With this plumbing in mind, can you see how B and T cells enter the lymph node? That's right, they can enter via the high endothelial venules by pushing their way between the high endothelial cells. There is also another way lymphocytes can enter the lymph node. Do you see it? Of course -- through the lymph. After all, lymph nodes are "dating bars," positioned along the route the lymph takes on its way to be reunited with the blood. Lymphocytes actively engage in "bar hopping," and are carried from node to node by the lymph. Although lymphocytes have two ways to gain entry to a lymph node, they only exit via the lymph -- those high endothelial venules don't let lymphocytes back into the blood.

Since lymph nodes are places where antigen and lymphocytes meet, we need to discuss how antigen enters a node. Dendritic cells stationed out in the tissues can be stimulated by battle cytokines to enter the lymph and carry antigens they have acquired at the battle scene into the secondary lymphoid organs for presentation to T cells. So this is one way that antigen can enter the lymph node: as "cargo" aboard APCs. In addition, antigen that has been opsonized by complement or antibodies can be carried by the lymph into the lymph node where it can be phagocytosed by macrophages for presentation to Th cells, or captured by follicular dendritic cells for presentation to B cells.

From these plumbing considerations, you probably have guessed that one function of a lymph node is as a "lymph filter." When lymph enters the node, it percolates through holes in the marginal sinus (sinus is a fancy word for cavity), through the cortex and paracortex, and finally into the medullary sinus where it is collected and leaves the node.

The walls of the marginal sinus are lined with macrophages that are tasked with cleaning up the lymph by phagocytosis. Other macrophages are found in the part of the lymph node called the paracortex. The high endothelial venules are also located in the paracortex, so lymphocytes pass through this region of the node when they arrive from the blood. In fact, T cells tend to accumulate in the paracortex, being retained there by adhesion molecules. This accumulation of T cells makes good sense, because macrophages and dendritic cells are also found in the paracortex, and of course, one object of this game is to get T cells together with these APCs.

If a helper T cell encounters its cognate antigen presented by an APC, it will be activated and will begin to proliferate in the paracortex. This proliferation phase lasts a few days. Most of these newly-activated Th cells will then exit the node via the lymph, recirculate through the blood, and re-enter lymph nodes via high endothelial venules. This process of recirculation is fast -- it generally takes less than a day -- and it is extremely important. Four major ingredients are required in order for the adaptive immune system to make antibodies: APCs to present antigen to Th cells, Th cells with receptors that recognize the presented antigen, opsonized antigen displayed by follicular dendritic cells, and B cells with receptors that recognize the antigen. Early in an infection, there are not a lot of any of these ingredients around, and naive B and T cells just circulate through the secondary lymphoid organs at random, checking for a match to their receptors. So the probability is pretty small that the rare Th cell that recognizes a particular antigen will arrive at the very same lymph node that is being visited by the rare B cell with specificity for that same antigen. However, if activated Th cells first proliferate to build up their numbers, and then recirculate to lots of lymph nodes and other secondary lymphoid organs, the Th cells with the right stuff get "spread around," so they have a much better chance of encountering those B cells for which they can provide help.

When the recirculating Th cells enter a node where their cognate antigen is being presented, they will be re-stimulated. Some of the re-stimulated Th cells will proliferate more and recirculate again to spread the help even further. Other re-stimulated Th cells will move to the lymphoid follicles of the lymph node to provide help to needy B cells, and still others will exit the blood to provide cytokine help to warriors doing battle in the tissues.

Killer T cells are also activated in the paracortex of the lymph node if they find their cognate antigen presented by virus-infected macrophages or dendritic cells, and if they receive cytokine help (e.g., IL-2) from activated Th cells. Once activated, CTLs proliferate and recirculate. Some of these CTLs re-enter secondary lymphoid organs and begin this cycle again, whereas others exit the blood at sites of infection to kill virus-infected cells.

B cells also engage in cycles of activation, proliferation, circulation, and re-stimulation, but there are still some mysteries surrounding just where and how virgin B cells are first activated. The most recent evidence indicates that B cells, which have encountered their cognate antigen displayed on follicular dendritic cells, migrate to the border of the lymphoid follicle where they meet activated T cells that have migrated there from the paracortex. It is during this "meeting" that B cells receive the co-stimulation they require for activation. Both B and T cells then enter the lymphoid follicles and the B cells begin to proliferate. Many of these newly-made B cells exit the lymphoid follicle via the lymph. Some become plasma cells that take up residence in the spleen or bone marrow where they pump out tons of antibodies. Others recirculate through the lymph and blood, and re-enter secondary lymphoid organs. As a result, activated B cells are spread around to many secondary lymphoid organs where, if they are re-stimulated in lymphoid follicles, they can undergo somatic hypermutation and class switching.

The frantic activity in germinal centers is usually over in about three weeks. By this time, the invader has been repulsed, and most of the opsonized antigen has been "picked" from the dendritic cells by B cells -- you remember that antigen is taken into the B cell after it has been bound by the BCR. At this point most B cells will have left the follicles or will have died there, and the areas that once were germinal centers will look much more like primary lymphoid follicles.

In summary, lymph nodes act as "lymph filters" in which antigen is picked up by APCs and follicular dendritic cells. These nodes also provide a concentrated environment of APCs, T cells, and B cells in which naive B and T cells can be activated, and experienced B and T cells can be re-stimulated. In lymph nodes, naive B and T cells can mature into cells that produce antibodies (B cells), provide cytokine help (Th cells), and kill infected cells (CTLs). In short, the lymph node can do it all.

As everyone knows, lymph nodes that drain sites of infection tend to swell. For example, if you have a viral infection of your upper respiratory tract (e.g., influenza), the cervical nodes in your neck may become swollen. You understand now that this swelling is due in part to the proliferation of lymphocytes in the node. In addition, cytokines from T cells in an active lymph node recruit additional macrophages which tend to plug up the medullary sinus. As a result, fluid is retained in the node, causing further swelling. When the invader has been defeated, there is no longer sufficient antigen to maintain B and T cells in an activated state. At this point, most B and T cells die from exhaustion or from lack of stimulation, but some of them go back to a resting state to provide a reservoir of memory cells that can quickly be re-activated if the virus attacks again. And of course, the swelling in your lymph nodes goes away.

PEYER'S PATCHES

Back in the late seventeenth century, a Swiss anatomist, Johann Peyer, noticed that embedded in the villi-covered cells that line the small intestine are patches of smooth cells. We now know that these "Peyer's patches" are examples of mucosal-associated lymphoid tissues (MALT) which function as secondary lymphoid organs.

Peyer's patches have high endothelial venules through which lymphocytes can enter, and, of course, there are outgoing lymphatics that drain lymph away from these tissues. However, unlike lymph nodes, there are no incoming lymphatics that bring lymph into Peyer's patches. Here's a diagram that shows one of the smooth cells that is part of a Peyer's patch:

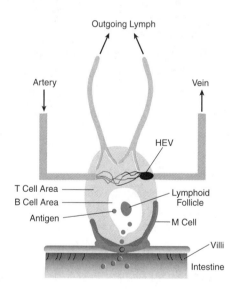

So if there are no incoming lymphatics, how does antigen enter this secondary lymphoid organ? That smooth cell that crowns the Peyer's patch -- the one that doesn't have "hairs" (villi) on it -- is called an "M" cell. It is a specialized cell that transports antigen from the interior (lumen) of the intestine into the Peyer's patch. To sample the contents of the intestine, M cells take in "sips" of antigen and enclose them in vesicles called endosomes that are roughly similar to

the phagosomes of macrophages. These endosomes are transported across the M cell, and their contents are then spit out the other side. So, whereas lymph nodes sample antigens from the lymph, Peyer's patches sample antigens from the intestine -- and they do it by transporting the antigen <u>through</u> the M cell!

Antigen that has been collected by M cells can be carried by the lymph to the lymph nodes that drain the Peyer's patches. In addition, if the collected antigen is opsonized by complement or antibodies, it can be captured by follicular dendritic cells in the lymphoid follicles that are below the M cells. In fact, except for its unusual method of acquiring antigen, a Peyer's patch is quite similar to a lymph node, with high endothelial venules to bring in T and B cells and special areas where these cells congregate.

THE SPLEEN

The final secondary lymphoid organ on our tour is the spleen. The spleen is located between an artery and a vein, and it functions as a blood filter. As with Peyer's patches, there are no lymphatics that bring lymph into the spleen. However, in contrast to lymph nodes and Peyer's patches, where entry of B and T cells from the blood occurs only via high endothelial venules, the spleen is like an "open-house party" in which everything in the blood is invited to enter. Here is a schematic diagram of one of the filter units that make up the spleen:

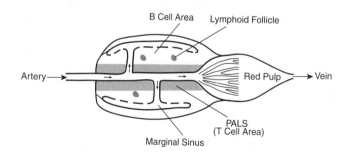

When blood enters from the splenic artery, it is diverted out to the marginal sinuses from which it percolates through the body of the spleen before it is collected into the splenic vein. The marginal sinuses are lined with macrophages that clean up the blood by phagocytosing cell debris and foreign invaders. As they ride along with the blood, B cells and T cells are temporarily retained in different areas -- T cells in a region called the periarteriolar lymphocyte sheath (PALS) that surrounds the central arteriole, and B cells in the region between the PALS and the marginal sinuses. Once activated by APCs in the PALS, T cells move into the lymphoid follicles, and give help to B cells that have recognized their cognate antigen -- you know the drill.

By now, I'm sure you have caught on to what Mother Nature is doing here. Each secondary lymphoid organ is strategically positioned to intercept invaders that enter the body by different routes. If the skin is punctured and the tissues becomes infected, an immune response is generated in the lymph nodes that drain those tissues. If you eat contaminated food, an immune response is generated in the Peyer's patches that line your intestine. If you are invaded by blood-borne pathogens, your spleen is there to filter them out and to initiate an immune response. If you are attacked via your respiratory tract, another set of secondary lymphoid organs that includes your tonsils is there to defend you.

Not only are the secondary lymphoid organs strategically positioned, they react by mobilizing weapons that are appropriate to the kinds of invaders they are most likely to encounter. For example, Peyer's patches specialize in Th cells that secrete a Th2 profile of cytokines, and B cells that secrete IgA antibodies -- weapons that are perfect to defend against intestinal invaders. In contrast, if you are attacked by bacteria from a splinter in your toe, lymph that contains bacteria and bacterial debris will find its way to the lymph node behind your knee. That node will produce Th1 cells and B cells that secrete IgG antibodies -- weapons that are ideal for defending against bacteria.

LYMPHOCYTE TRAFFICKING

So far, we have talked about the secondary lymphoid organs in which B and T cells meet to do their activation thing, but we haven't said much about how these cells know to go there. Immunologists call this process "lymphocyte trafficking," and as you'll see, the traffic patterns for virgin and experienced lymphocytes are different. So let's start with the virgins.

T cells begin life in the bone marrow and are educated in the thymus -- lots more on this part in the next lecture. When they emerge from the thymus, virgin T cells express on their surfaces a mixture of cellular adhesion molecules that function as "world-wide passports" for travel to any of the secondary lymphoid organs. For example, virgin T cells have a molecule called L-selectin on their surfaces that can bind to its adhesion partner, GlyCAM-1, which is found on the high endothelial venules of lymph nodes. This is their "lymph node passport." Virgin T cells also express the integrin $\alpha 4\beta 7$, whose adhesion partner, MadCAM-1, is found on the high endothelial venules of Peyer's patches and the lymph nodes that drain the tissues around the intestines (the mesenteric lymph nodes). So this integrin is their passport to the gut region. Because of these adhesion molecules, inexperienced T cells are encouraged to circulate through all of the secondary lymphoid organs. In these organs, they pass through fields of antigen presenting cells in the T cell areas. If they are not activated, they re-enter the blood either via the lymph or directly (in the case of the spleen), and continue to recirculate, making a complete circuit every twelve to twenty-four hours. If a T cell does not encounter its cognate antigen presented by an MHC molecule, it eventually dies, lonely and unsatisfied, by apoptosis. In contrast, those lucky T cells that do encounter their antigen are activated in the secondary lymphoid organs. These are now "experienced" T cells.

Experienced T cells carry passports too, but they are "restricted passports," because, during activation, expression of certain cellular adhesion molecules on the T cell surface is increased, while expression of others is decreased. This modulation of cellular adhesion molecule expression is not random -- there's a plan here. In fact, the cellular adhesion molecules that activated T cells express depend on where these T cells were activated. For example, T cells activated in a Peyer's patch will express high levels of $\alpha 4\beta 7$ (the gut-specific integrin), and low levels of L-selectin (the more general, high endothelial venule adhesion molecule). As a result, these T cells tend to return to Peyer's patches. Thus, when activated T cells recirculate, they usually exit the blood and re-enter the same type of secondary lymphoid organ in which they originally encountered antigen. This restricted traffic pattern makes perfect sense. After all, there is no use having T cells recirculate to the lymph node behind your knee if your lower intestine is inflamed, because you ate some bad food. Certainly not. You want those T cells to get right back to the gut to be re-stimulated and to provide help. So by equipping activated T cells with restricted passports, Mother Nature insures that the T cells go where they are needed, be it to Peyer's patches, lymph nodes, or tonsils.

Now, of course, you don't want T cells to just go round and round. You also want them to exit the blood at sites of inflammation, so they can kill virus-infected cells or provide cytokines that amplify the immune response and recruit even more warriors from the blood. To make this happen, experienced T cells also carry passports (adhesion molecules) that allow them to exit the blood at sites of inflammation. These T cells use the same "roll, sniff, stop, exit" technique that neutrophils use to squeeze between the endothelial cells that line blood vessels and to exit the blood into inflamed tissues. For example, T cells that gained their experience in the mucosa express the integrin molecule αEβ7, which just happens to have as its adhesion partner an addressin molecule that is expressed on inflamed mucosal blood vessels. So adhesion molecules on the surfaces of experienced T cells allow them to leave the blood and enter tissues exactly where the battle is going on.

In summary, naive T cells have passports that allow them to visit all secondary lymphoid organs, but not sites of inflammation. This traffic pattern brings the entire collection of virgin T cells into contact (in the secondary lymphoid organs) with invaders that may have entered the body at any point, and greatly increases the probability that the virgin T cells will be activated. The reason that virgin T cells don't carry passports to battle sites is that they couldn't do anything there anyway -- they must be activated first.

In contrast to virgin T cells, experienced T cells have restricted passports that encourage them to return to the same type of secondary lymphoid organ as the one in which they gained their experience. By recirculating preferentially to the kind of tissue in which they first encountered antigen, T cells are more likely to be re-stimulated or to find CTLs and B cells that have encountered the same invader and need their help. In addition, activated Th cells and CTLs have passports that allow them to exit the blood at sites of infection, so that CTLs can kill infected cells and Th cells can provide appropriate cytokines to direct the battle. This marvelous system of cellular adhesion molecules insures delivery of the right weapons to the sites where they are needed.

B cell trafficking has not been studied as extensively as T cell trafficking, but the two processes seem rather similar. Like virgin T cells, virgin B cells also have general passports that admit them to the complete range of secondary lymphoid organs. However, experienced B cells don't tend to be as migratory as experienced T cells. Most just settle down in secondary lymphoid organs and in the bone marrow, produce antibodies, and let these antibodies do the traveling.

WHY MOTHERS KISS THEIR BABIES

Have you ever wondered why mothers kiss their babies? It's something they all do, you know. Most of the "barn yard" animals kiss their babies too, although in that case we call it licking. I'm going to tell you why they do it.

The immune system of the newborn human is not very well developed. In fact, production of IgG antibodies doesn't really begin until a few months after birth. Fortunately, IgG antibodies in the mother's blood can cross the placenta into the fetus's blood, so the newborn has this "passive immunity" from the mother to help tide it over. The newborn can also receive another type of passive immunity: IgA antibodies from mother's milk. During lactation, plasma B cells migrate to the mother's breasts and produce IgA antibodies that are secreted into the milk. This works great, because most pathogens that the baby encounters enter through the mouth and nose, travel to the baby's intestines, and cause diarrhea. By drinking mother's milk that is rich in IgA, the baby's alimentary tract is coated with antibodies that can intercept these pathogens.

When you think about it, however, a mother has been exposed to many different pathogens during her life, and the antibodies she makes to most of them will not be of any use to the infant. For example, it is likely that the mother has antibodies to the Epstein Barr virus that causes mononucleosis, but babies probably won't be exposed to this virus until they start kissing. So wouldn't it be great if the mother could somehow provide antibodies that recognize the very pathogens that the baby is encountering -- and not provide antibodies that the baby has no use for? Well, that's exactly what happens! When a mother kisses her baby, she "samples" those pathogens that are on the baby's face -- the very ones that the baby is about to ingest. These samples are taken up by the mother's secondary lymphoid organs like the tonsils, and memory B cells specific for those pathogens are re-stimulated. These B cells then migrate to the mother's breasts where they produce just those antibodies that the baby needs!

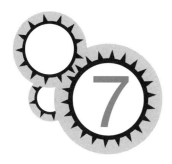

7 TOLERANCE INDUCTION AND MHC RESTRICTION

REVIEW

Let's begin our review of the material we covered in the last lecture by discussing the life of a B cell. These cells are born and educated in the bone marrow, and because of the adhesion molecules they display on their surfaces, virgin B cells travel to secondary lymphoid organs like lymph nodes and Peyer's patches looking for their cognate antigens. If they are unsuccessful, they continue circulating through the blood, lymph, and secondary lymphoid organs until they either find their cognate antigens or die of neglect. In the lymphoid follicles of the secondary lymphoid organs, the lucky B cell that finds the antigen to which its receptors can bind will migrate to the border of the lymphoid follicle. There, if it receives the required co-stimulation from an activated helper T cell, the B cell will be activated, and will proliferate to produce many more B cells with the same antigen specificity.

All this activity converts a primary lymphoid follicle, which is just a loose collection of follicular dendritic cells and B cells, into a "germinal center" in which B cells proliferate and mature. In the germinal center, B cells may switch isotypes, so they can produce IgA, IgG, or IgE antibodies, and they may undergo somatic hypermutation to increase the average affinity of their receptors for antigen. Most of these B cells become plasma cells and travel to the spleen, bone marrow, and secondary lymphoid organs, where they produce antibodies. Others recirculate to secondary lymphoid organs that are similar to the one in which they were activated. There they can amplify the response by being re-stimulated to proliferate some more. Still other B cells go back to the resting state in the spleen or bone marrow to function as memory cells.

T cells are also born in the bone marrow, but they then journey to the thymus to be educated -- the subject of today's lecture. Virgin Th cells that survive this educational experience travel though the blood, and under the influence of adhesion molecules, enter secondary lymphoid organs. If a Th cell does not encounter its cognate antigen displayed by an APC in the T cell zone, it exits the organ via the lymph or the blood, and visits other secondary lymphoid organs in search of its antigen.

If, while visiting a secondary lymphoid organ, a Th cell does find its cognate antigen displayed by class II MHC molecules on an antigen presenting cell (e.g., a dendritic cell), it will be activated and will proliferate. Most of the progeny exit the secondary lymphoid organ and travel through the lymph and the blood. These "experienced" Th cells have adhesion molecules on their surfaces that encourage them to re-enter the same type of secondary lymphoid organ in which they were activated (e.g., a Peyer's patch vs. a peripheral lymph node). This recirculation following initial activation and proliferation functions to spread the Th cells around to the more than a thousand secondary lymphoid organs where B cells or CTLs may be waiting for their help. Recirculating Th cells can also exit the blood vessels that run through sites of inflammation. There the Th cells can amplify the immune response by providing cytokines that strengthen the reaction of the innate and adaptive systems to the invader, and that recruit even more immune system cells from the blood.

Virgin CTLs also circulate through the blood, lymph, and secondary lymphoid organs. They can be activated if they encounter their cognate antigen displayed by class I MHC molecules on the surface of an antigen presenting cell in the T cell zones of secondary lymphoid organs. Like Th cells, they can proliferate and recirculate to secondary lymphoid organs to be re-stimulated, or they can leave the circulation and enter inflamed tissues to kill cells infected with viruses or other parasites.

In summary, virgin B and T cells are equipped with adhesion molecules that promote travel to all secondary lymphoid organs, but which do not allow travel to inflamed tissues. As a result, the entire repertoire of TCRs and BCRs is brought together in secondary lymphoid organs where the probability is highest that they will encounter their cognate antigens in an environment appropriate for activation. Once activated, B and T cells receive restricted passports to travel back to the same type of secondary lymphoid organ in which they were originally activated, and to exit the blood at sites of infection.

In the last lecture, we talked in some detail about three representative secondary lymphoid organs: a lymph node, a Peyer's patch, and the spleen. B and T cells enter lymph nodes from the blood (by passing between specialized high endothelial cells) or via the lymph. Antigen and APCs bearing antigen enter lymph nodes via lymph drained from tissues, so this organ functions as a lymph filter that intercepts invaders. In contrast, antigen is transported into the Peyer's patches through specialized M cells that sample antigen in the intestine. This antigen can either interact with B and T cells that have entered the Peyer's patches via high endothelial venules or can travel with the lymph to nearby lymph nodes that drain the Peyer's patch. Thus, the Peyer's patch is a secondary lymphoid organ that is designed to deal with pathogens attempting to breach the intestinal mucosal barrier. Finally, we talked about the spleen, a secondary lymphoid organ that is quite different from either a lymph node or a Peyer's patch in that it has no incoming lymphatics and no high endothelial venules. As a result of this "plumbing," antigen and lymphocytes must enter the spleen via the blood. This construction makes the spleen an ideal blood filter that intercepts blood-borne pathogens.

So the secondary lymphoid organs play critical roles in immunity. Not only do they create an environment in which antigen, antigen presenting cells, and lymphocytes can get together to initiate an immune response, they also are strategically located to intercept invaders that may breach the physical barriers and enter tissues, blood or mucosa.

SELF TOLERANCE AND MHC RESTRICTION

The subject of this lecture is one of the most exciting in all of immunology. Part of that excitement arises because, although a huge amount of research has been done on tolerance and MHC restriction, there are still many unanswered questions. What really makes this topic so exciting, however, is that it is so important: T cells must "learn" not to recognize our own "self" antigens as dangerous, for otherwise we would certainly die of autoimmune disease. In addition, T cells must be "restricted" to recognize self MHC, so that the attention of T cells is focused on MHC-peptide complexes and not on unprocessed antigen. Nobel Prizes await the immunologists who finally discover how T cells are taught these two important lessons.

Perhaps the major problem in understanding tolerance and MHC restriction is that it is technically very difficult to follow T cells around as they are educated to be tolerant of self and restricted to recognize self MHC molecules. What you'd like to do is to introduce a model "self" antigen into an animal (mice are quite popular), and observe how T cells that have receptors for this antigen are tolerized or restricted. However, because T cell receptors are so diverse, only a tiny fraction of the T cells in a mouse will have receptors that recognize a given antigen (usually fewer than one T cell in a million). So following those rare T cells around in the crowd of T cells that don't recognize your favorite antigen is really tough.

To increase the number of T cells that respond to a given antigen, two methods have been devised, neither of which is without flaws. The first method involves the use of "super antigens." These are proteins that cause the activation of a relatively large fraction (usually 5-25%) of the helper T cells in a mouse. There are two sources of superantigens: toxins produced by bacteria and proteins encoded by viruses. In both cases, superantigens work by binding to the variable region of the TCR and to the class II MHC molecule, "clamping" them together.

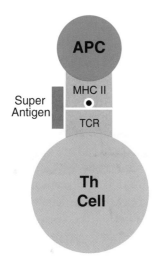

This superantigen "clamp" makes the binding between the MHC molecule and the TCR so strong that essentially every T cell that happens to have this particular variable region will be activated. As you can imagine, having 25% of your Th cells activated all at once might be a problem, and in fact, the super antigen encoded by a common bacterium, *Staph aureus*, can cause toxic shock syndrome and food poisoning by hyperactivating the immune system. Although super antigens were all the rage a few years ago, this tool is less popular now, because immunologists recognize that the way a T cell receptor interacts with a super antigen is quite different from the "normal" interaction between TCR and MHC-peptide that we have discussed in earlier lectures.

The second tool immunologists have used to follow T cells around is a mouse that makes TCRs with only one specificity. As you probably know, transgenic mouse technology has progressed to the point where you can wipe out just about any gene you wish and replace it with another one. All you need are lots of mice and lots of money. Anyway, what immunologists have done is to wipe out the gene segments that normally are mixed and matched to make a TCR, and to replace them with a pre-assembled TCR gene that recognizes some particular protein (e.g., a protein from a chicken) presented by either class I or class II MHC. As a result, every Th cell or CTL in these TCR transgenic mice will recognize the chicken protein, and that makes it much easier to follow these T cells through their education process. However, as you will see during this lecture, the number of TCRs that a T cell expresses on its surface changes with time as the cell matures and is educated. So far, the TCRs in these transgenic mice

don't behave that way -- they are expressed at a certain level and that's it. So when interpreting an experiment that uses these mice, you have to ask whether the results that are obtained might be influenced by the timing and the level of TCR expression.

THE THYMUS

T cells learn tolerance of self in two places. The first is in the thymus, and this kind of tolerance is usually called "central" tolerance. The second is outside the thymus, and this is called "peripheral" tolerance. The thymus is a very mysterious organ. Although quite a bit is known about what goes on inside the thymus, relatively little is known about how cells and antigen gain access to this organ.

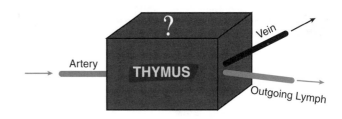

You will notice right away that, like the spleen, the thymus has no incoming lymphatics, so cells enter the thymus from the blood. However, in contrast to the spleen, which welcomes anything that is in the blood, entry of cells into the thymus is quite restricted -- although immunologists don't know yet what the "password" is. Immature T cells from the bone marrow are presumed to enter the thymus from the blood, somewhere in the middle of the thymus. However, exactly how these cells exit the blood is not understood, because the high endothelial cells that allow lymphocytes to exit the blood into secondary lymphoid organs are missing from the thymus. Antigens are also thought to enter from the blood, but again, the rules that govern their entry are unclear.

What is known is that the T cells which enter the thymus from the bone marrow are "nude" -- that is, they don't express CD4, CD8, or a TCR. After entering, these cells make their way to the outer region of the thymus (the "cortex"), and begin to proliferate.

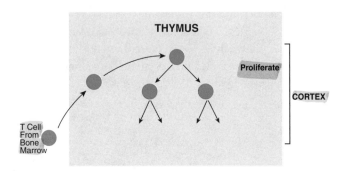

About this time, some of the cells start to rearrange the gene segments that encode the β and α chains of the TCR. If these rearrangements are successful, the T cell begins to express low levels (i.e., relatively few molecules) of the TCR and its associated, accessory proteins. As a result, these formerly-nude cells are soon "dressed" with CD4, CD8, and TCR molecules. Because these T cells express both CD4 and CD8 co-receptor molecules, they are called double positive (DP) cells.

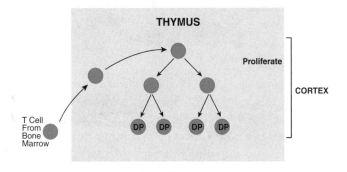

During this "reverse striptease," another important change takes place. When the T cell was nude, it was resistant to death by apoptosis, because it expressed no Fas antigen (which can trigger death when ligated) and it expressed high levels of Bcl-2 (a cellular protein that protects against apoptosis). In contrast, in its double-positive state, the T cell expresses high levels of Fas on its surface and it produces very little Bcl-2. As a result, it is quite vulnerable to signals that can trigger apoptosis. It is in this highly vulnerable state that the T cell will be tested for tolerance of self and MHC restriction. If it fails either test, it will be killed.

MHC RESTRICTION

Immunologists still are not sure of the order in which these two exams are taken, so for the sake of discussion, I'll assume that the exam for MHC restriction precedes the exam for tolerance of self. The process of testing T cells for MHC restriction is usually referred to as "positive selection." The "examiners" here are epithelial cells in the cortical region of the thymus, and the exam question that the T cells must answer is: "Do you recognize self MHC molecules expressed on the cortical epithelial cell?" The correct answer is, "Yes, I do!" for if the TCR does not recognize any of the self MHC molecules, the T cell dies.

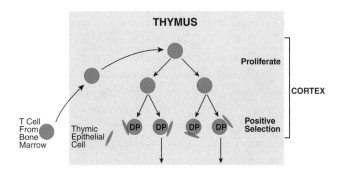

When I say "self" MHC, I simply mean those MHC molecules expressed by the person (or mouse) who "owns" this thymus. Yes, this does seem like a "no brainer" -- that my T cells would be tested in my thymus on my MHC molecules -- but immunologists like to emphasize this point by saying "self MHC."

The MHC molecules on the surface of the cortical epithelial cells are actually loaded with peptides, so what the TCR really recognizes is self MHC plus peptide. These peptides are a "sampling" of all the proteins that are normally made by the cortical epithelial cells (class I display) or a "sampling" of all the proteins that are present in the thymic environment at that moment (class II display). Those lucky T cells that have TCRs that can recognize self MHC plus peptide proceed to the second test.

THE LOGIC OF MHC RESTRICTION

Let's pause here for a moment and ask an important question: Why do T cells need to be tested to be sure that they can recognize peptides presented by self MHC? After all, most humans complete their lifetimes without ever seeing "foreign" MHC molecules (e.g., on a transplanted organ), so MHC restriction can't involve discriminating between your MHC molecules and mine. No, MHC restriction has nothing to do with foreign vs. self -- it has to do with "focus." As we discussed in Lecture Four, we want the system to be set up so that T cells focus on antigen that is presented by MHC molecules. Because T cell receptors are made by mixing and matching gene segments, they are incredibly diverse. As a result, it is certain that in the collection of TCRs expressed on T cells, there will be many that recognize "native," unpresented antigen just as B cell receptors do. These T cells must be eliminated, otherwise the wonderful system of antigen presentation by MHC molecules won't work. So the reason positive selection (MHC restriction) is so important is that it sets up a system in which all mature T cells will have TCRs that recognize antigen presented by MHC molecules.

CENTRAL TOLERANCE INDUCTION

The second test in the thymus is for tolerance of self, and this is frequently referred to as "negative selection." The exam question here is, "Do you recognize MHC plus self peptide?" and the correct answer is, "No way!" T cells with receptors that do recognize the combination of MHC and self peptide fail this exam, and die by apoptosis. The cells that administer this test are different from those that test for positive selection. Whereas the positively selecting cells are "real" thymus cells that have been present in the thymus since embryonic development, the negatively selecting cells are dendritic cells that have migrated to the thymus from the bone marrow. These thymic dendritic cells reside mainly in the central region of the thymus called the medulla.

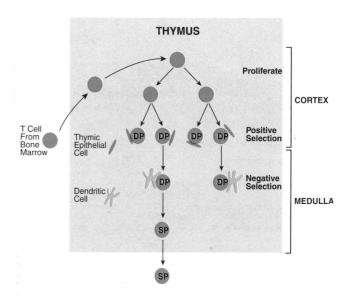

Most of my students are not too thrilled about exams that last more than an hour, so I thought you might be interested to know that these two exams take about two weeks! We're talking major exams here -- a life and death struggle. The final result of all this testing is a T cell with receptors that will not react against self antigens presented by MHC molecules on thymic dendritic cells, but which will recognize self MHC-peptide complexes presented by thymic epithelial cells.

The "thymic graduates" that pass these tests express high levels (i.e., many molecules) of the T cell receptor on their surfaces, and either the CD4 or CD8 co-receptor, but not both -- so they are called single positive (SP) cells. Each day in the thymus of a young person, about 60 million double positive cells are tested, but only about 2 million single positive cells exit the thymus -- so roughly 3% of the "candidates" pass these exams. The rest die by apoptosis, and are quickly eaten by macrophages in the thymus.

THE LOGIC OF TOLERANCE INDUCTION

Clearly the reason for this second exam is to eliminate T cells that could react against our own "self" antigens. If such self-reactive T cells were not eliminated, autoimmune disease could result: Th cells could help B cells make antibodies that would tag our own molecules as dangerous, and CTLs could be produced that would attack and destroy our own cells. This much is obvious, but there is an interesting subtlety here. To introduce it, let me ask you a question: For T cells undergoing tolerance induction in the thymus, what is the functional definition of "self antigen"?

It turns out that the only "self" that really matters to a T cell taking this exam are the self peptides that happen to be displayed on the negatively-selecting, thymic dendritic cells at the time the exam is taking place. Mature thymic dendritic cells only live for a few days in the thymus. As a result, they only present what you might call "current" self antigen. This is really smart, because if foreign antigens were to reach the thymus (as they certainly can during an infection), dendritic cells could take up these antigens and use them for testing, just as if they were authentic "self" antigens. As a result, any maturing T cells that recognized the invader would be "deleted" for as long as thymic dendritic cells continued to present the foreign antigens. Thus, the short lifetime of dendritic cells protects against this possibility, and allows T cells to be examined only on "new material." As a result, once foreign antigens associated with an infection have been eliminated, freshly-made dendritic cells will no longer present foreign antigen as self, and T cells that can recognize the invader will again survive negative selection.

THE RIDDLE OF MHC RESTRICTION AND TOLERANCE INDUCTION

If you've been paying close attention, you may be wondering how any T cells could possibly pass both exams. After all, to pass the test for MHC restriction, TCRs must be able to recognize MHC plus self peptide. Yet to pass the tolerance test, TCRs must not be able to recognize MHC plus self peptide. So the riddle is: How can the same T cell receptor possibly mediate both positive selection (MHC restriction) and negative selection (tolerance induction)? In fact, it is even more complicated than that, because once T cells have been educated in the thymus, their TCRs must then be able to signal activation when they encounter invaders presented by MHC molecules. So how does MHC-peptide engaging the same TCR result in these three, very different outcomes -- positive selection, negative selection, and activation? It's quite a riddle.

Unfortunately, I can't answer this riddle (otherwise I'd be on my way to Sweden), but I can tell you what the current thinking is about MHC restriction and tolerance induction. Immunologists believe that the

events leading to MHC restriction and tolerance induction are similar to those that we discussed earlier for activation of T cells: cell-cell adhesion, TCR clustering, and co-stimulation. The current thinking is that in the thymus, positive selection (survival) of T cells with receptors that recognize self MHC results from a relatively weak interaction between TCRs and MHC-self peptide displayed on thymic epithelial cells. Negative selection (death) of cells with TCRs that recognize self antigens in the thymus is induced by a strong interaction between TCRs and MHC-self peptide expressed on bone marrow-derived, thymic dendritic cells. Activation of T cells after they leave the thymus results from a strong interaction between TCRs and MHC-peptide displayed by professional antigen presenting cells.

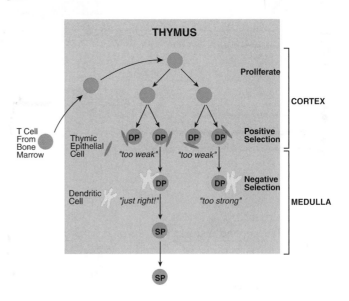

The riddle, of course, is just what makes the effect of these three interactions of MHC-peptide with the T cell receptor so different -- life, death, activation. One key element appears to be the properties of the cell that "sends" the signal. In the case of MHC restriction, this is a thymic epithelial cell. For tolerance induction, the cell is a bone marrow-derived dendritic cell. For activation, the "sender" is a specialized antigen presenting cell. These cells are very different, and it is likely that they differ in the cellular adhesion molecules they express, and in the number of MHC-peptide complexes they display on their surfaces. These differences could dramatically influence the "strength" of the signal that is sent through the T cell receptor. In addition, these three cell types are likely to express different mixtures of co-stimulatory molecules, and co-stimulatory signals could change the character of the signal that results from TCR-MHC-peptide engagements. Finally, recent evidence suggests that the enzymes that cut up proteins for class II display in thymic epithelial cells are different from the enzymes that do the cutting in thymic dendritic cells. Thus, there is the possibility that, at least for class II, the collections of peptides involved in positive and negative selection are different.

Not only are the cells that send the signals different, but the "receiver" (the T cell) also may change between exams. For example, it is known that the number of TCRs on the surface of the T cell increases as the cell is educated. It is also possible that the "wiring" within the T cell changes as the T cell matures, so that the "receptor engaged" signal is processed in different ways. These differences in TCR density and wiring could influence the "interpretation" of the signals sent by the three types of sender cells.

So although many of the pieces of the puzzle probably have been found, immunologists still have not been able to assemble them into a consistent story. It is very likely, however, that this important riddle will soon be solved.

TOLERANCE BY IGNORANCE

Although the mechanisms involved in central tolerance induction are not well understood, most T cells with TCRs that recognize self peptides in the thymus are eliminated. However, central tolerance is certainly not foolproof. If it were, every single TCR would have to be tested on every possible self antigen in the thymus -- and that's a lot to ask. For T cells with receptors that have a high affinity for self antigens that are abundant in the thymus, the probability is very high that they will be deleted. However, T cells with receptors that have a low affinity for self antigens, or that recognize self antigens which rarely are found in the thymus, are less likely to be negatively selected -- they may just slip through the "cracks" of central tolerance induction. Fortunately, the system has been set up to deal with this possibility.

In the last lecture we discussed lymphocyte trafficking, and you learned that virgin lymphocytes are free to circulate through the blood, lymph, and secondary lymphoid organs, but that they are not allowed out into the tissues. As a rule, those self antigens that are abundant in the secondary lymphoid organs where

virgin lymphocytes are activated are also abundant in the place where T cells are tolerized, the thymus. Therefore, as a result of the traffic pattern followed by virgin T cells, most T cells that could be activated by abundant self antigens found in secondary lymphoid organs will already have been eliminated by seeing that same abundant self antigen in the thymus.

In contrast, T cells whose receptors recognize antigens that are relatively rare in the thymus may escape deletion there. However, these antigens are usually also present at such low concentrations in the secondary lymphoid organs that the density of MHC-peptide complexes will be insufficient to activate these T cells. Thus, although rare self antigens are present in the secondary lymphoid organs, and although T cells have receptors that can recognize them, these T cells remain functionally "ignorant" of their presence, because the antigens are too rare to trigger activation. So lymphocyte traffic patterns play a key role not only in insuring the efficient activation of the adaptive immune system, but also in preserving tolerance of self antigens.

PERIPHERAL TOLERANCE

Of course, the traffic patterns of virgin T cells aren't perfect, and some virgins do stray from the beaten path and venture into the tissues. To deal with this situation, there is a third level of protection against autoimmunity -- peripheral tolerance.

The problem with virgin T cells that violate the traffic laws is that they may encounter antigens that are too rare in the thymus to trigger negative selection, but which are quite abundant out in the tissues -- abundant enough to activate the T cell. For example, there are abundant self antigens that are only found in the heart or the kidney. Such "organ-specific" antigens are usually not present at any appreciable level in the thymus, so T cells with receptors that recognize these self antigens will breeze right through negative selection.

Fortunately, the activation requirements for virgin T cells are quite stringent. Not only must virgin T cells encounter antigen presented by a cell on which there is a high density of MHC-peptide complexes (so that their TCRs can be crosslinked), but they must also receive co-stimulatory signals from the cell that is presenting the antigen. That's where professional antigen presenting cells come in. These cells have a high density of MHC complexes on their surfaces and they also express co-stimulatory molecules like B7 that are required for T cell activation -- that's why they're professionals. In contrast, "ordinary cells" like heart and kidney cells generally don't express high levels of MHC proteins or don't express co-stimulatory molecules, or both. As a result, a virgin T cell with TCRs that recognize a kidney antigen could go right up to a kidney cell, and not be activated by it. In fact, it's even better than that, because usually when a T cell recognizes its cognate antigen on a cell, but does not receive the appropriate co-stimulatory signals, that T cell is "neutered." Immunologists say the cell is "anergized." It looks like a T cell, but it can no longer perform. In many cases, cells that are anergized eventually die, so peripheral tolerance induction can result in either anergy or death (deletion).

TOLERANCE DUE TO ACTIVATION-INDUCED DEATH

Okay, so what if a T cell escapes deletion in the thymus, breaks the traffic laws, ventures out into the tissues, and happens to find its cognate antigen displayed by MHC molecules at a high enough density to crosslink its receptors on a cell that just happens to express enough B7 co-stimulatory protein to activate the T cell. What then? Well, all is not lost, because there is yet another "layer" of tolerance protection that can help out in this unlikely situation. It is called activation-induced cell death. Here's how it works:

Once an invader has been vanquished, it is very important that mechanisms exist which will turn the immune response off. For example, T cells must be continuously re-stimulated to avoid apoptotic death, so once the invading antigens have been eliminated, most T cells die off. But there is another way that T cells can be "deleted" when they are no longer needed. T cells that have been re-stimulated multiple times during an invasion express the Fas protein on their surfaces. When it is engaged by its ligand, FasL, the Fas protein can trigger the cell to commit suicide by apoptosis. However, activated CTLs already express the Fas ligand -- that is one of the ways they kill their target cells. So these "old" CTLs end up expressing both FasL and Fas, and this deadly combination causes them to die by apoptosis. In addition, old helper T cells -- ones that have been repeatedly re-stimulated -- become targets

for CTL killing when they begin to express the Fas protein. The end result is that "worn out" T cells are deleted.

Getting rid of old T cells by activation-induced cell death makes perfect sense. After all, most invasions by viruses or bacteria result in acute infections that either are quickly dealt with by the immune system (in a matter of days or weeks) or that overwhelm the immune system and kill you. So there is no reason to have activated T cells survive for a long period to deal with an acute infection. In contrast, if a T cell is activated by a self antigen out in the tissues, the result is usually chronic inflammation in which T cells are stimulated over and over by the self antigens. In this situation, self-reactive T cells "wear out" and die by activation-induced apoptosis. It is as if the immune system senses that this kind of chronic activation "ain't natural," and does away with the offending T cells.

In summary, induction of T cell tolerance is multilayered. No single mechanism of tolerance induction is 100% efficient, but because there are multiple mechanisms, autoimmune diseases are relatively rare. T cells with receptors that recognize antigens that are abundant in the secondary lymphoid organs usually are efficiently deleted in the thymus. Self antigens that are rare enough in the thymus to allow self-reactive T cells to escape deletion usually are also too rare to activate virgin T cells in the secondary lymphoid organs. Thus, because of their restricted traffic pattern, virgin T cells normally remain ignorant of rare self antigens. In those cases where virgin T cells do venture outside the blood-lymph-secondary lymphoid organ system, they generally encounter tissue-specific antigens in a context that leads to anergy or death, not activation. Finally, those rare T cells that are activated by recognizing self antigens in the tissues usually die from chronic re-stimulation.

B CELL TOLERANCE

Immunologists once thought that it might not be necessary to delete B cells with receptors that recognize self antigens, because the T cells that would be needed to "help" these self-reactive B cells would already have been killed or anergized. In that case, B cells would be "covered" by T cell tolerance. However, as it became clear that B cells could be activated without T cell help, it was realized that there must be some mechanism(s) for tolerizing B cells. Although B cell tolerance has not been as well studied as T cell tolerance, there do seem to be many similarities between tolerance induction in B and T cells, and for this reason, I will only touch lightly on B cell tolerance.

It is now believed that B cells can be tolerized where they are born -- in the bone marrow. This would be the B cell equivalent of "central" tolerance induction. When "young" B cells encounter abundant self antigens in the bone marrow they die by apoptosis. Fortunately, B cells in the bone marrow are exposed to the same abundant self antigens that are found in the secondary lymphoid organs where virgin B cells are activated. Therefore, as with T cells, the traffic pattern of virgin B cells helps "protect" them from encountering abundant self antigens that would not have been present in the bone marrow during central tolerance induction. There are also mechanisms that can tolerize B cells that break the traffic laws. Virgin B cells that venture into the tissues can be anergized or deleted if they recognize their cognate antigen, but do not receive T cell help. In addition, B cells that are chronically stimulated by self antigens eventually die by apoptosis (activation-induced apoptosis). Thus, B cells are subject to mechanisms of peripheral tolerance induction that are similar, but probably not identical, to those that tolerize T cells outside the thymus.

MAINTENANCE OF B CELL TOLERANCE IN GERMINAL CENTERS

You may be wondering whether B cells undergoing somatic hypermutation might end up with receptors that can recognize self antigen. If they did, these B cells could produce antibodies that would recognize our own antigens and cause autoimmune disease. Fortunately, it turns out that this usually doesn't happen, and the reasons are quite interesting.

B cells in the germinal center are very "fragile." Unless they receive "rescue" signals, they die by apoptosis. In this sense, germinal center B cells resemble the fragile T cells that undergo MHC restriction and tolerance induction in the thymus. The signals required to rescue B cells from death in the germinal center are the same as those required to activate B cells in the first place: recognition of cognate antigen in a form that crosslinks BCRs, and co-stimulatory signals from helper T cells. B cells seem to need these two rescue sig-

nals more or less continuously while they are in the germinal center.

If a B cell mutates so that its receptors recognize a self antigen, it is very unlikely to find (and be rescued by) that self antigen advertized on follicular dendritic cells. After all, FDCs only display antigens that have been opsonized, and self antigens are usually not opsonized by complement, because the innate immune system doesn't recognize self antigens as "dangerous." Recent experiments also indicate that for a B cell to be rescued from death in the germinal center, not only must its BCRs be crosslinked by antigen, but its complement receptors (which function as "co-receptors") must also engage complement fragments that are opsonizing the antigen. This double requirement for BCR and complement receptor crosslinking probably explains why humans who lack a functional complement system do not have germinal centers.

So the first problem that self-reactive B cells face in the germinal center is the lack of complement-opsonized self antigen on follicular dendritic cells. But they have another problem -- lack of co-stimulation -- and the reason for this is even more interesting. After Th cells have been activated in the T cell zones of secondary lymphoid organs, they migrate to the lymphoid follicles to give help to B cells. This help involves co-stimulation in which the CD40L protein on the T cell binds to the CD40 protein on the B cell. However, while this interaction between CD40L and CD40 is taking place, the engaged CD40L is rapidly taken into the interior of the Th cell. Pretty soon, the Th cell doesn't have enough CD40L left on its surface to co-stimulate the B cell -- it "runs out of gas." At this point, the Th cell must be re-stimulated if production of CD40L is to be increased, so that more surface CD40L will be available to provide co-stimulation. But the Th cell is no longer in the T cell zone where the APCs that originally provided stimulation reside. So how does the Th cell get re-stimulated? Well, when B cells bind their cognate antigen on follicular dendritic cells, it is internalized, cut into fragments, and presented on class II MHC molecules. In addition, activated B cells also express B7 -- the co-stimulatory molecule that Th cells need to be re-stimulated. So in the lymphoid follicle, B cells can act as antigen presenting cells to re-stimulate Th cells. Now the neat part.

What is the relationship between the B cell's cognate antigen, and the antigen it presents to the Th cell? That's right. The B cell presents a fragment of its cognate antigen to the Th cell. So to have this mutual activation thing between B and T cells work, the B cell and T cell must be looking at parts of the same antigen. Now, if the B cell hypermutates so that its BCRs bind to and present a new antigen (e.g., a self antigen), the Th cell needed to co-stimulate the B cell will not recognize this antigen -- because it's no longer the Th cell's cognate antigen. As a result, the B and T cells will not be able to cooperate to keep each other stimulated.

Because B cells require T cell help to survive in the germinal center, this interdependence of T and B cells helps keep B cells "on track" as they go through hypermutation. So self tolerance is preserved during B cell hypermutation for two reasons: the lack of complement-opsonized self antigen required for efficient BCR crosslinking, and the lack of co-stimulation from germinal center Th cells for B cells that recognize self antigen.

EPILOGUE

At this point you should have a good overall view of how the immune system is designed to work in healthy individuals. In the next two lectures, we will explore the role that the immune system plays in disease.

A SUMMARY FIGURE

T cell tolerance is a multilayered process in which several "levels" of tolerance-inducing mechanisms insure that, for most humans, autoimmunity never happens.

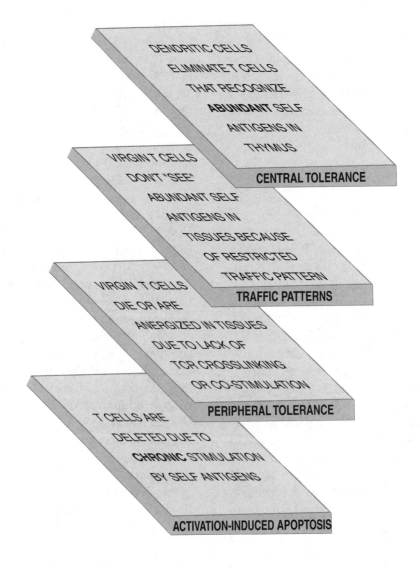

PART II

The Immune System in Disease

8

IMMUNOPATHOLOGY--
THE IMMUNE SYSTEM GONE WRONG

REVIEW

Let's review the last lecture on tolerance and MHC restriction. In that lecture, we discussed what is probably the most important riddle left to be solved by immunologists: How can the same T cell receptor mediate positive selection (MHC restriction), negative selection (tolerance induction), and activation? This riddle has not been solved, but here's the current thinking:

In the thymus, positive selection of T cells with receptors that recognize self MHC results from a relatively weak interaction between TCRs and MHC-self peptide displayed on thymic epithelial cells. This weak interaction is enough to insure that TCRs are "focused" on antigen that is presented by MHC molecules, so that recognition is restricted to presented antigens, not "native" antigens. In contrast, negative selection (death) of cells with TCRs that recognize self antigens in the thymus is induced by a strong interaction between TCRs and MHC-self peptide expressed on bone marrow-derived, thymic dendritic cells. Finally, activation of T cells after they leave the thymus results from a strong interaction between TCRs and MHC-peptide displayed by professional antigen presenting cells.

The important point here is that the interactions that lead to these three very different outcomes are between the TCR and MHC-peptide on three very different types of cells. These cells can be expected to express different adhesion molecules, different co-stimulatory molecules, and even different cytokines, so the outcome of each of these interactions could depend heavily on the cell type with which the T cell interacts. In addition, T cells may "learn from experience": Their signaling pathways may change as they are educated and mature.

Although the mechanisms are not completely understood, the end result of the thymic experience is that only about 3% of the T cells that enter selection exit from the thymus. Those T cells that survive have receptors that do not recognize MHC plus peptides derived from self antigens that are relatively abundant in the thymus. Of course, many T cells that exit the thymus have receptors that will recognize foreign peptides presented by MHC -- that's the whole idea of this game -- but some of them also have receptors that can recognize relatively rare self antigens that are not abundant enough in the thymus to efficiently delete T cells. So although thymic tolerance is pretty good, it isn't the whole story. To take care of T cells that slip through thymic selection, several mechanisms exist <u>outside</u> the thymus that back up thymic tolerance induction. These mechanisms are lumped together under the heading of "peripheral tolerance."

One way of dealing with T cells that escape deletion in the thymus is to restrict the trafficking of virgin T cells to blood, lymph, and secondary lymphoid organs. Most self antigens that are abundant in the secondary lymphoid organs also are abundant in the thymus, so T cells with receptors that could recognize these self antigens will already have been deleted there. On the other hand, self antigens that are not abundant enough in the thymus to efficiently delete T cells usually are present in secondary lymphoid organs at concentrations too low to activate potentially self-reactive T cells. Therefore, many virgin T cells remain ignorant of the existence of their cognate self antigens, simply because there isn't enough antigen around to trigger activation.

So the traffic pattern of naive T cells works together with thymic tolerance induction to protect us from self-reactive T cells that could cause autoimmune disease. However, not all virgin T cells are law-abiding, and some will leave their normal circulation pattern and wind up in the tissues. To deal with these "law breakers," Mother Nature has a few more tricks up her sleeve. For T cells to be activated, they must first recognize their cognate MHC-peptide combination at a high enough concentration to trigger activation. Fortunately, most cells in the tissues don't express high enough levels of MHC-peptide to activate naive T cells.

Virgin T cells must also receive co-stimulatory signals from the cell that presents the antigen, and whereas antigen presenting cells in the secondary lymphoid organs are specialized to provide this co-stimulation, your everyday cell out in the tissues is not. To take advantage of this fact, T cells are programmed so that when they do recognize antigen in the absence of adequate co-stimulation, they are anergized or killed. Thus, even if cells in the tissues happen to express enough MHC-self peptide complexes to adequately crosslink T cell receptors, they generally don't express the co-stimulatory molecules required to rescue T cells from death or anergy. Finally, even in the rare event that T cells are activated by cells in the tissues that express adequate levels of MHC-self peptides and co-stimulatory molecules, these T cells usually die due to chronic stimulation by self peptides.

The picture you should have is that none of the mechanisms for tolerizing T cells is foolproof -- they all are a little "leaky." However, because there are multiple levels of tolerance inductions to catch potentially self-reactive T cells, the whole system works very well, and relatively few humans suffer from serious autoimmune disease.

B cell tolerance is less well studied than T cell tolerance, but the available data indicate that tolerance induction in B cells is also multilayered. Unlike T cells, which have a separate organ, the thymus, in which central tolerance is induced, B cells that react against relatively abundant self antigens are eliminated where they are born, in the bone marrow. Virgin B cells mainly traffic through the blood, lymph, and secondary lymphoid organs where they are exposed to the same abundant self antigens that they "viewed" in the bone marrow. Naive B cells that wander out of this traffic pattern usually don't encounter sufficient self antigen in a form that can crosslink their BCRs. In addition, virgin B cells whose receptors are crosslinked by self antigen in tissues usually don't receive the co-stimulatory signals required for activation -- and crosslinking without co-stimulation can anergize or kill B cells. Finally, if B cells are chronically re-stimulated (e.g., by self antigens in the tissues), they eventually die by apoptosis, adding yet another layer of protection against self-reactivity.

IMMUNOPATHOLOGY

So far, we have focused on the "good" that the immune system does in protecting us from infection. Occasionally, however, the immune system "goes wrong" -- sometimes with devastating consequences. In this lecture we will examine four categories of diseases in which the immune system plays a major role in producing the damaging effects (the pathology) of the disease. First, we will discuss examples of diseases in which the normal functioning of the immune system results in pathological consequences. Next, we will examine diseases that result when the systems that usually control the immune response don't function properly. Then we will discuss autoimmune diseases caused by a breakdown in the mechanisms that normally insure tolerance of self. Finally, we will focus on diseases that stem from immunodeficiencies, both genetic and acquired.

PATHOLOGICAL CONDITIONS CAUSED BY A NORMAL IMMUNE RESPONSE

Tuberculosis is an excellent example of a disease whose pathological consequences are the result of normal immune system function. Tuberculosis is usually contracted by inhaling microdroplets containing the TB bacterium (*Mycobacterium tuberculosis*) that are generated by the cough of an infected individual. When these bacteria are taken into the lungs, they are confronted by macrophages that are stationed there to intercept invaders that enter via the respiratory tract.

From Lecture One, you remember that when a macrophage encounters a bacterium, the macrophage first engulfs it in a pouch (vesicle) called a phagosome. This vesicle is then taken inside the macrophage where it fuses with another vesicle called a lysosome, which contains powerful chemicals that can destroy the bacterium.

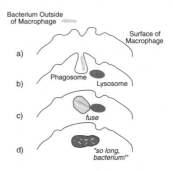

Unfortunately, in the case of the tuberculosis bacterium, the macrophage bites off more than it can chew, because the TB bacterium is able to resist destruction by lysosomal chemicals and escape from the phago-lysosome into the cytoplasm of the macrophage. Now the bacterium is in heaven, because the cytoplasm contains all the nutrients it needs to grow and multiply. Eventually, many newly-minted bacteria burst out of the macrophage, killing it, and go on to infect other macrophages in the area. As the macrophage dies by necrosis, the contents of its lysosomal vesicles are released into the tissues of the lung. This causes tissue damage, and initiates an inflammatory reaction.

The struggle between macrophages and the TB bacteria results in the production of battle cytokines that can hyperactivate macrophages in the lung. Once hyperactivated, macrophages can better deal with TB bacteria, because the killing power of their lysosomal weapons increases. Some battle cytokines can also recruit additional immune system cells to the scene, increasing the inflammatory reaction.

Macrophages and the cells they recruit sometimes win this battle and eliminate the invading bacteria. In other cases, it's a fight to a draw, and a state of chronic inflammation results in which the bacteria are kept in check, but macrophages continue to be killed, and the lungs continue to be damaged by the inflammatory reaction. So in a TB infection, the pathology of the disease results from macrophages doing exactly what they are supposed to do -- engulf invaders.

Sepsis is another disease that is due to the immune system doing all the right things. Sepsis is a rather generic term that describes the symptoms that can result from a systemic infection. Such an infection is usually caused by bacteria that enter the blood stream when the physical barriers that are our first line of defense are breached. For sepsis to occur in a healthy individual, a large number of bacteria usually must be introduced. This could occur, for example, as a result of bacterial escape from an abscess or other formerly-localized infection. In patients with a suppressed immune system (e.g., during chemotherapy for cancer), much smaller quantities of bacteria are required.

Although both Gram-negative and Gram-positive bacteria can cause sepsis, the classic culprits are Gram-negative bacteria like *E. coli* that have LPS (lipopolysaccharide) as a component of their cell walls, and which also shed this molecule into their surroundings. As we discussed in Lecture Two, LPS is a potent

danger signal that can activate macrophages and NK cells. These two cells then work together in a positive feedback loop that increases their activation states, and that produces cytokines which recruit neutrophils and additional macrophages and NK cells from the blood.

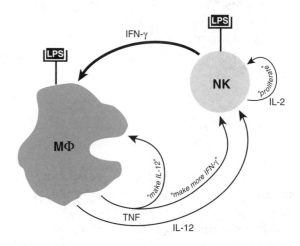

Helper T cells of the Th1 type are also recruited, and these "quarterback" cells set up their own positive feedback loops with macrophages that increase the level of macrophage activation, and influence uncommitted Th0 cells from the blood to become Th1-type cells.

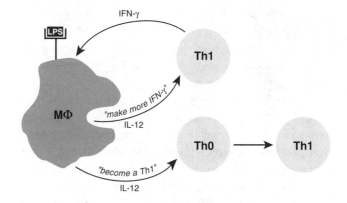

Under normal conditions, the function of these positive feedback loops is to amplify the immune response, so that the innate and adaptive systems can respond quickly and strongly to a localized infection. However, in a "full-body" infection, in which bacteria carried by the blood enter tissues everywhere, this amplified response can get out of hand. TNF secreted by activated macrophages can cause blood vessels to become "leaky," so that fluid escapes from the vessels into the surrounding tissues. In extreme cases, the decrease in blood volume due to system-wide leakage can cause a drop in blood pressure that results in shock (septic shock) and heart failure. So sepsis and septic shock can result when the positive feedback loops that normally allow the immune system to react strongly and quickly to an invasion cause an over-reaction to a system-wide infection.

DISEASES CAUSED BY DEFECTS IN IMMUNE REGULATION

Roughly 20% of the U.S. population suffers from allergies to common environmental antigens (allergens) that are either inhaled or ingested. These normally non-pathogenic antigens, which are constantly in contact with our respiratory or gastrointestinal mucosa, are largely ignored by the immune systems of non-allergic individuals, who respond weakly to these antigens, and who produce mainly Th1 helper cells and low levels of IgG antibodies. In striking contrast, allergic individuals (called "atopic" individuals) produce mainly allergen-specific Th2 cells and large quantities of IgE antibodies. Indeed, the concentration of IgE antibodies in the blood of atopic individuals can be 1,000- to 10,000-fold higher than in the blood of non-atopic people. It is this defect in the regulation of helper T cell types (favoring Th2 cells over Th1 cells) and the resultant over-production of IgE antibodies in response to otherwise innocuous environmental antigens that are largely responsible for allergic reactions.

In Lecture Three, we discussed the interaction of IgE antibodies with mast cells. Since mast cell degranulation is a central event in many allergic reactions, let's take a moment to review this concept. When atopic individuals are first exposed to an allergen (e.g., pollen) they produce large amounts of IgE antibodies directed against the allergen. Mast cells have receptors on their surfaces that can bind to the Fc region of IgE antibodies, so that after the initial exposure, mast cells will have large numbers of IgE molecules attached to their surfaces. On a second or subsequent exposure, the allergen can crosslink the IgE molecules on the mast cell surface, dragging the Fc receptors together. This clustering of Fc receptors signals mast cells to "degranulate" -- to dump the granules that normally are stored

inside them into the tissues in which they reside.

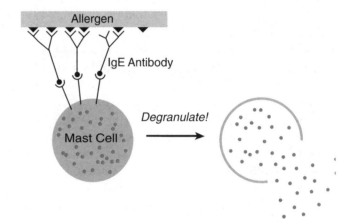

Mast cell granules contain histamine and other powerful chemicals and enzymes that can cause the symptoms which atopic individuals are intimately familiar with. However, mast cells are only one of the cells involved in allergic reactions. Another white blood cell, the basophil, also has receptors for IgE antibodies, and crosslinking of these receptors can lead to basophil degranulation. A third cell that is important in allergic reactions (especially delayed reactions) is the eosinophil. This white blood cell is found predominately in tissues beneath skin and mucosa. Recent evidence indicates that eosinophils also have receptors for IgE antibodies, and that crosslinking of these receptors may be one of the signals that triggers eosinophil degranulation during an allergic reaction. Of course, mast cells, basophils, and eosinophils were not invented by Mother Nature just to annoy allergic people. These cells, with their ability to degranulate "on command," provide a defense against those parasites that are too large to be phagocytosed by professional phagocytes.

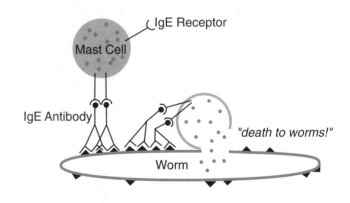

So IgE antibodies are the bad guys in allergic reactions -- but what causes some people to make IgE antibodies to antigens like pollen, while others make IgG antibodies in response to exactly the same antigen? You remember from Lecture Five that helper T cells can be influenced by the environment in which they are re-stimulated to secrete various cytokines, and that these cytokine profiles can be polarized toward the production of a Th1 or Th2 subset of cytokines.

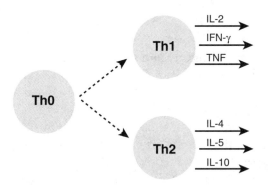

In turn, B cells undergoing class switching are influenced to switch to production of IgA, IgG, or IgE antibodies, depending on the cytokine environments in germinal centers where class switching takes place. For example, a germinal center that is populated with Th1 cells usually will produce B cells that make IgG antibodies, because Th1 cells secrete IFN-γ which drives the IgG class switch. In contrast, B cells tend to switch to IgE production if they switch isotypes in germinal centers that contain Th2 cells which secrete IL-4 and IL-5. So the decision to produce either IgG or IgE antibodies in response to an allergen will mainly depend on the type of helper T cells that are present in the secondary lymphoid organs that intercept the allergen. Indeed, helper T cells from allergic individuals show a much stronger bias toward the Th2 type than do Th cells from normal, non-atopic people.

Okay, so atopic individuals produce IgE antibodies because their allergen-specific helper T cells tend to be of the Th2 type. But how do they get that way? The answer to this question is not known for certain, but I'll tell you what some of the latest thinking is. Many immunologists now believe that a bias toward either Th1- or Th2-type helper T cells is usually established early in childhood, and in some cases, even before birth.

The fetus inherits half its genetic material from its mother and half from its father. As a result, the fetus is really a "transplant" that expresses many paternal antigens to which the mother's immune system is not tolerant. Since the placenta is the interface between the mother and the fetus, measures must be taken to avoid having maternal CTLs and NK cells attack cells in the placenta that express paternal antigens. The Th1 subset of helper cells secretes TNF that helps activate NK cells, and IL-2 that causes NK cells and CTLs to proliferate. So it would be advantageous for the survival of the fetus to bias maternal Th cells away from the Th1 cytokine profile that favors a "cellular" response, and toward a Th2 profile that favors a more benign, antibody response. In turns out, in fact, that the placenta produces relatively large amounts of IL-4 and IL-10 -- the major cytokines that influence Th cells to become Th2 cells.

So to protect the fetus, the placenta secretes cytokines that impair the mother's cellular response -- and the same cytokines also have a strong influence on fetal helper T cells. As a result, most humans are born with a strong bias toward a Th2 cytokine profile. Obviously, this bias does not last a lifetime, and eventually most people end up with a more balanced population of Th1 and Th2 cells. One event that probably helps establish a Th cell balance is infection at an early age with microbes (viruses or bacteria) that normally elicit a dominant Th1 response. Immunologists suspect that microbial infections may also be important in producing a Th1 response to allergens. Here's how this is thought to work:

Immunologists hypothesize that if a microbial infection strongly "deviates" the immune response of a young child toward a Th1 type at the same time that the child encounters an allergen (say, pollen), the Th response to that allergen will also be deviated toward the Th1 type. Once this deviation takes place, feedback mechanisms will tend to lock in the Th1 response to that allergen, and memory T cells will be generated that remember not only the allergen but also their Th1 response to it. Once a large number of biased memory cells is built up, it is difficult to reverse this bias, so early exposure to infectious diseases may be critical in establishing a normal response to environmental allergens. This "immune deviation" hypothesis is consistent with the increase in the incidence of allergies and the corresponding decrease in the incidence of microbial infections (e.g., tuberculosis) seen in developed countries.

In addition to environmental factors (e.g., early

exposure to infectious diseases), heredity clearly plays a large part in susceptibility to allergies. For example, if one identical twin suffers from allergies, the probability is about 50% that the second twin will also be atopic. The genes that confer susceptibility to allergies have been difficult to identify, because there seem to be many of them, and because they differ from atopic individual to atopic individual. It is known, for example, that people who are allergic to certain allergens are more likely to have inherited particular class II MHC genes than are non-atopic people. The thinking here is that the MHC molecules encoded by these genes may be especially efficient at presenting these allergens. In addition, some atopic individuals are known to produce mutant forms of the IgE receptor. It is hypothesized that these mutant receptors send an unusually strong signal when crosslinked, resulting in secretion of abnormally high levels of IL-4 by mast cells, favoring the production of IgE antibodies. Finally, mutations have been detected in the regulatory (promoter) region of the IL-4 gene, and these mutations might also increase the amount of IL-4 that atopic individuals produce.

The best current synthesis of this information is that the immunological basis for allergies is a defect in immune regulation in which allergen-specific helper T cells are strongly polarized toward the Th2 cytokine profile, resulting in the production of allergen-specific, IgE antibodies. The genes a person inherits can make him or her more or less susceptible to allergies, and exposure to environmental factors such as microbial infections may influence whether susceptible individuals become atopic.

AUTOIMMUNE DISEASE

Autoimmune disease results when a breakdown in the mechanisms meant to preserve tolerance of self is severe enough to cause a pathological condition. Rather than expend a huge amount of biological "energy" on a foolproof system in which each B and T cell is carefully checked for tolerance of self, Mother Nature evolved a multilayered system in which each layer includes mechanisms that should weed out most self-reactive cells, with lower layers catching cells that slip through tolerance induction in the layers above. This multilayered system works very well, but occasionally "mistakes are made," and the system breaks down.

Indeed, roughly 5% of Americans suffer from some form of autoimmune disease.

Autoimmune disorders can result from obvious genetic defects. For example, most autoimmune diseases are chronic disorders that involve repeated stimulation of self-reactive lymphocytes. In normal people, this is controlled by "activation-induced cell death" in which T cells that are repeatedly stimulated express the Fas protein. This makes them targets for killing by CTLs or for self-induced apoptosis. Humans who have genetic defects in either Fas or FasL lack this layer of tolerance protection, and their T cells refuse to die when chronically stimulated by self antigens. The resulting diseases, autoimmune lymphoproliferative syndrome and Canale-Smith syndrome, have as their pathologic consequences massive swelling of lymph nodes, production of antibodies that recognize self antigens, and the accumulation of large numbers of T cells in the secondary lymphoid organs.

Although some autoimmune disorders result from genetic defects, immunologists believe that the majority of autoimmune diseases result when the layers of tolerance inducing mechanisms fail to eliminate self-reactive cells in genetically normal individuals. Thus, it appears that the potential for autoimmune disease is the price we must pay for having T and B cell receptors that are so diverse that they can recognize essentially any invader.

The latest thinking is that for autoimmunity to occur, at least three conditions must be met. First, an individual must express MHC molecules that can efficiently present a peptide derived from the target self antigen. Therefore, the MHC molecules you inherit can play a major role in determining susceptibility to autoimmune disease. For example, only about 0.2% of the U.S. population suffers from juvenile diabetes, yet for Caucasian Americans who inherit two particular types of class II MHC genes, the probability of being diabetic is increased about twenty-fold.

The second requirement for autoimmunity is that the afflicted person must produce T, and in some cases B cells that have receptors which recognize the self antigen. Because TCRs and BCRs are made by a mix and match strategy, the repertoire of receptors that one individual expresses will be different from that of every other individual, and will change with time as lymphocytes die and are replaced. Even the collections of TCRs and BCRs expressed by identical twins will be different. Therefore, it is largely by chance that a person will produce lymphocytes whose receptors can recognize a particular self antigen.

MOLECULAR MIMICRY

So for autoimmune disease to occur, a person must have MHC molecules that can present self antigens and T cells with receptors that can recognize these presented antigens -- but this is not enough. In addition, there must be environmental factors that lead to the breakdown of the normal tolerance mechanisms that are designed to eliminate self-reactive lymphocytes. For years, physicians have noticed that autoimmune diseases frequently follow bacterial or viral infections, and immunologists believe that microbial attack may be one of the key environmental factors that trigger autoimmune disease. Now, clearly a viral or bacterial infection cannot be the whole story, because for most people these infections do not result in autoimmunity. However, in conjunction with a genetic predisposition (e.g., type of MHC molecules inherited) and lymphocytes with potentially self-reactive receptors, a microbial infection may be the "last straw" that leads to autoimmune disease. Immunologists' current favorite hypothesis to explain why infections might lead to a breakdown in self tolerance is called "molecular mimicry." Here's how this is thought to work:

Lymphocytes have BCRs or TCRs that recognize their cognate antigen. It turns out, however, that this is almost never a single antigen. Just as one MHC molecule can present a large number of peptides that have the same general characteristics (length, binding motif, etc.), a TCR or a BCR usually can recognize several antigens. Generally, a TCR or BCR will have a high affinity for one or a few of these cognate antigens, and relatively lower affinities for the others. As a result of this promiscuity, TCRs and BCRs usually "cross react" with several antigens.

According to the molecular mimicry hypothesis, T or B cells whose receptors recognize certain microbial antigens will be activated in the normal course of an immune reaction to the microbial invasion. If, however, these receptors happen to cross react with self antigens, an autoimmune response to the self antigens can result. It is presumed that before the microbial infection, these potentially self-reactive lymphocytes had not been activated because the affinities of their receptors for self antigen were too low to trigger activation, or because the restricted traffic patterns of virgin lymphocytes never brought them into contact with self antigens under conditions that would allow activation. However, once activated in response to a cross-reacting microbial antigen, these self-reactive lymphocytes can now do real damage.

Animal models of human autoimmune diseases have been very useful for understanding which immune system players are involved, which self antigens are targets of the immune reaction, and which microbial antigens might be involved in the molecular mimicry that triggers disease. Typically, these models involve animals that have been bred to be exquisitely susceptible to autoimmune disease, or animals whose genes have been altered to make them susceptible. One lesson learned from animal models and from humans is that it is unlikely that a single environmental antigen is responsible for a given autoimmune disease, because TCRs which recognize self antigens usually cross react with multiple environmental antigens (e.g., viral or bacterial proteins).

INFLAMMATION AND AUTOIMMUNE DISEASE

Although molecular mimicry may be responsible for the activation of lymphocytes that previously had been "ignorant" of self antigens, there must be more to the story. After all, when self-reactive T cells activated by a mimic reach the tissues, they are in a precarious situation. To avoid apoptotic death by "neglect," they must be continuously re-stimulated, and if they encounter self antigens in an environment that does not provide both sufficient receptor crosslinking and co-stimulation, they will be anergized or deleted.

As you remember, the innate system usually gives "permission" for the adaptive system to function. An important part of this permission involves the activation of antigen presenting cells by inflammatory cytokines such as IFN-γ and TNF which are secreted by cells of the innate system in response to an attack. Once activated, APCs (e.g., macrophages) will express the MHC and co-stimulatory molecules that are required to re-stimulate T cells which have entered the tissues. So when lymphocytes venture out into the tissues to help with a battle that the innate system is already fighting, re-stimulation is not a problem. However, for a lymphocyte that recognizes a self antigen that the innate system does not recognize as dangerous, the tissues can be a very inhospitable place, because the self-reactive lymphocyte usually will not find the co-stimulation necessary for its survival.

The bottom line is that it is not enough for a microbe to activate self-reactive T cells by mimicry. There must also be an inflammatory reaction going on in the same tissues that express the self antigen. Otherwise it is unlikely that self-reactive T cells would exit the blood into these tissues, and if they did, that they would be re-stimulated.

So the scenario most immunologists favor for the initiation of autoimmune disease is: An individual who is genetically susceptible is attacked by a microbe that activates T cells whose receptors just happen to cross react with a self antigen. Simultaneously, an inflammatory reaction takes place in the tissues where this self antigen is expressed. This inflammation could be caused either by the mimicking microbe itself, or by another, unrelated infection or trauma. As a result of this inflammatory reaction, APCs will be activated that can pick up self antigen from damaged tissues, and use it to re-activate self-reactive T cells. In addition, cytokines generated by the inflammatory response can upregulate class I MHC expression on normal cells in the tissues, making these cells better targets for destruction by self-reactive CTLs.

EXAMPLES OF AUTOIMMUNE DISEASE

Autoimmune diseases are usually divided into two groups: organ-specific and multi-system diseases. Let's look at examples of both types, paying special attention to the self antigens against which the immune response is thought to be directed, and to the environmental antigens that may be involved in molecular mimicry.

An important example of an organ-specific autoimmune disease is insulin-dependent diabetes mellitus. In this disease, the targets of autoimmune attack are the insulin-producing "β cells" of the pancreas. Although antibodies produced by self- reactive B cells may participate in the chronic inflammation that contributes to the pathology of this disease, it is currently believed that the initial attack on the β cells is mediated by CTLs.

Clearly, there are genetic factors that help determine susceptibility to diabetes, since the probabil-

ity that both identical twins will have this autoimmune disease is about 50%. In diabetes, destruction of the insulin-producing cells in the pancreas usually begins months or even years before the first symptoms of diabetes appear. Fortunately, antibodies to β cell antigens are produced very early in the disease, and these antibodies are now being used to identify relatives of diabetic patients who may also be afflicted. Unfortunately, no strong candidates have emerged for environmental factors that might trigger the initial attack on β cells.

Myasthenia gravis is an autoimmune disease that results when self-reactive antibodies bind to the receptor for an important neurotransmitter, acetylcholine. When the message that is normally carried by acetylcholine from nerve to muscle is not received (because the antibodies interfere with its reception), muscle weakness and paralysis can result. A region of one of the poliovirus proteins is similar in amino acid sequence to part of the acetylcholine receptor, so it is possible that a polio infection could provide a mimic that would activate lymphocytes whose receptors cross react with the acetylcholine receptor.

Multiple sclerosis is an inflammatory disease of the central nervous system that is thought to be initiated by self-reactive T cells. In multiple sclerosis, chronic inflammation destroys the myelin sheaths that are required for nerve cells in the brain to transmit electrical signals efficiently, causing defects in sensory inputs (e.g., vision) and paralysis. Macrophages recruited by cytokines secreted by T cells are thought to play a major role in causing this inflammation. At first there was a question as to how T cells could get into the brain to initiate this disease, but eventually it was discovered that activated T cells (but not virgin T cells) can cross the blood-brain barrier.

The presumed target of these T cells is a major component of the myelin sheath, myelin basic protein. T cells that have been isolated from multiple sclerosis patients can recognize a peptide derived from myelin basic protein as well as peptides derived from proteins encoded by herpes simplex virus or Epstein-Barr virus (the virus that causes mononucleosis). So a possible scenario is that when genetically susceptible individuals are infected with herpes virus or Epstein-Barr virus, they produce T cells that recognize proteins from these viruses. Some of these activated T cells may have receptors that cross react with myelin basic protein, and these activated T cells can cross the blood-brain barrier, lead the attack on the myelin sheaths, and cause multiple sclerosis. Of course not everyone who gets mononucleosis or a herpes infection gets multiple sclerosis, so exposure to microbial mimics is not the whole story. Indeed, multiple sclerosis is a disease in which there is clearly a strong genetic component: It is about ten times more probable that identical twins will share this disease than it is for non-identical twins to both be afflicted.

Pemphigus vulgaris is an autoimmune disease in which antibodies to a self protein (desmoglein I) on the surface of skin cells disrupt the adhesion between these cells and results in the formation of blisters on the skin. In fact, antibodies obtained from pemphigus patients can cause symptoms of the disease when injected into animals. Interestingly, a gene encoding one particular class II MHC molecule has so far only been found in patients with pemphigus, suggesting a strong role for MHC type in determining susceptibility to this disease.

Rheumatoid arthritis is a systemic autoimmune disease that is characterized by chronic inflammation of the joints. This inflammation is mediated mainly by macrophages (and the TNF they produce) that infiltrate the joints under the direction of self-reactive Th cells. Recent clinical trials have shown considerable improvement in patients treated with antibodies that inactivate TNF. One of the presumed targets of this autoimmune reaction is a cartilage protein, and T cells from arthritic patients can recognize both the cartilage protein and a protein encoded by the bacterium that causes tuberculosis. In fact, mice injected with *Mycobacterium tuberculosis* suffer from inflammation of the joints, suggesting, but not proving, that a mycobacterial infection may trigger rheumatoid arthritis in some patients. IgM antibodies that recognize and bind to the Fc region of IgG antibodies are also present in the joints of individuals with rheumatoid arthritis. These IgM-IgG antibody complexes help activate macrophages that have entered the joints, increasing the inflammatory reaction.

Finally, lupus erythematosus is a systemic autoimmune disease that affects about 250,000 people in the U.S., roughly 90% of whom are women. This disease can have multiple manifestations including a red rash on the forehead and cheeks (giving the "red wolf" appearance for which the disease is named), inflammation of the lungs, arthritis, kidney damage, hair loss, paralysis, and convulsions. Lupus is caused by a breakdown in both B and T cell tolerance that results in the production of IgG antibodies which recognize a wide range of self antigens including DNA, DNA-protein complexes, and RNA-protein complexes. The diversity of the self antibodies produced is thought to be reflected in the diversity of the disease symptoms.

Non-identical twins have about a 2% probability of both having lupus, whereas with identical twins, this probability increases about ten-fold. This indicates a strong genetic component to the disease, and multiple MHC and non-MHC genes have been identified, each of which seems to slightly increase the probability that a person will contract lupus.

Although no specific microbial infection has been associated with the initiation of lupus, mice that lack functional genes for Fas or Fas ligand exhibit lupus-like symptoms. This has led immunologists to speculate that lupus may result from a defect in activation-induced apoptosis, in which lymphocytes that should die due to chronic stimulation survive and cause the disease. However, in humans with lupus, no genetic defects in either Fas or FasL have been identified, so other proteins that are involved in the control of apoptosis may be defective in these patients.

In summary, autoimmune disease is thought to require three "ingredients": MHC molecules that are able to efficiently present self antigens, lymphocytes whose receptors can recognize self antigens, and additional environmental and/or genetic factors that allow mechanisms of tolerance induction to be circumvented. It is only when these three requirements are fulfilled that the pathological conditions associated with autoimmune disease will result. Although viral or bacterial infections may supply the environmental trigger for these diseases in susceptible individuals, it appears unlikely that any single microbe is responsible for any autoimmune disease.

ANTIGEN SPREADING

One of the reasons it has been so difficult for immunologists to identify environmental factors (e.g., the specific microbes) that trigger autoimmune disease is the phenomenon of "antigen spreading." When T or B cells are isolated from patients with autoimmune disease, collectively these lymphocytes usually recognize several, and in some cases many self antigens. What seems to be happening is that although autoimmunity may originally involve T or B cells that recognize a single, "initiating" self antigen, with time, other lympho-cytes that recognize additional self antigens will also be activated.

For example, in lupus it is suspected that the disease is initiated by T and B cells that recognize DNA coated with proteins (as DNA normally is in human cells) that is released from cells damaged by infection or trauma. Once started, the autoimmune response results in the recruitment of macrophages and additional lymphocytes. These recruited cells amplify the inflammatory response at the site by expressing cytokines such as IFN-γ and TNF that increase the efficiency of antigen presentation by macrophages and dendritic cells. The result is that other self antigens that have been released from damaged tissues, and which formerly were poorly presented due to inadequate MHC expression or inadequate co-stimulation, now can be presented efficiently enough to activate T cells that had previously ignored their existence. Consequently, the targets of self-reacting T cells "spread" from the initiating self antigen to other self antigens that originally were "quiet" enough to be ignored.

DISEASES DUE TO IMMUNO-DEFICIENCIES

Serious disease may result when our immune systems do not operate at full strength. Some immun-odeficiencies are caused by genetic defects that disable parts of the immune network. Others are "acquired" as the consequence of deliberate immunosuppression (e.g., during organ transplantation or chemotherapy for cancer) or disease (e.g., AIDS).

GENETIC DEFECTS LEADING TO IMMUNODEFICIENCY

We have already discussed several genetic defects that lead to immune system weakness. For example, individuals who are born with non-function-al CD40 or CD40L proteins are unable to mount a T cell-dependent antibody response, because T cells either cannot deliver or B cells cannot receive the all-impor-tant, co-stimulatory signal. We also discussed the importance of an intact complement system, and the fact that people who are born with defects in important complement proteins (e.g., C3), don't have germinal centers in their secondary lymphoid organs. The result of both the CD40-CD40L defect and the complement defect is that B cells secrete mainly IgM antibodies that have not affinity matured -- because class switching and somatic hypermutation take place in germinal centers and require co-stimulation by CD40L.

One extreme example of a genetic defect is severe combined immunodeficiency syndrome (SCIDS). It was because of this disease that the famous "bubble boy" had to be kept isolated in a pathogen-free environment. SCIDS patients lack functional B and T cells (that's the "combined" part). Although a number of different mutations can cause this condition, the best understood are defects in proteins required to carry out the gene rearrangements that produce functional B and T cell receptors. Without their receptors, lymphocytes are blind to the world around them and are totally use-less.

AIDS

Although genetic immunodeficiencies are rela-tively rare, millions of people suffer from immunodefi-ciencies that are acquired. By far the largest group of immunodeficient humans acquired their deficiency when they were infected with the AIDS virus. The symptoms that originally alerted physicians that they were dealing with a disease that had immunodeficien-cy as its basis was the high incidence of infections (e.g., pneumocystis carinii pneumonia) or cancers (e.g., Kaposi sarcoma) that are usually only seen in immuno-suppressed individuals. Soon, the virus that caused this immunodeficiency was isolated and named "human immunodeficiency virus 1" (HIV-1).

An HIV-1 infection begins very much like most other viral infections. Viruses in the initial inoculum enter cells, and use the cell's biosynthetic machinery to make many more copies of the virus. These newly-made viruses then burst out of the cell, and go on to infect other cells. So in the early stages of infection, the virus multiplies relatively unchecked while the innate system gives it its best shot, and the adaptive system is being mobilized. After a week or so, the adaptive sys-tem starts to kick in, and virus-specific B cells, helper T cells, and CTLs are activated, proliferate, and begin to do their thing. The "big gun" in most viral infections is the CTL, because each virus-infected cell may produce

10,000 new viruses, and CTLs can kill these cells before the viruses have a chance to multiply inside them.

So during this first, "acute" phase of an HIV-1 infection, there is a dramatic rise in the number of viruses in the body (viral load) followed by a marked decrease in the viral load as CTLs and antibodies go to work.

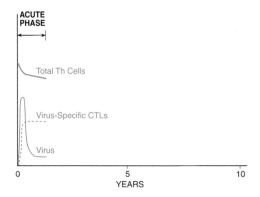

With many viruses (e.g., smallpox), the end result of the acute phase of a viral infection is "sterilization": All the invading viruses are destroyed, and memory B and T cells are produced to protect against a later infection with the same virus. There is some evidence that for a few, very lucky individuals, an HIV-1 infection may also end in sterilization. However, for the vast majority, infection with HIV-1 leads next to a "chronic" phase that can last for ten or more years. During this phase, a fierce struggle goes on between the immune system and the AIDS virus -- a struggle that, unfortunately, the virus always seems to win.

During the chronic phase of infection, viral loads decrease to low levels compared with those reached during the height of the acute phase, and the number of virus-specific CTLs and Th cells remains high -- a sign that the immune system is still trying hard to defeat the virus.

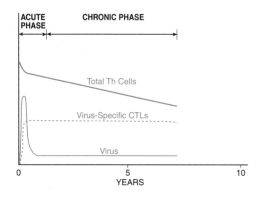

However, as the chronic phase progresses, the total number of Th cells slowly decreases, because these cells are killed as a consequence of the viral infection. Eventually there are not enough Th cells left to provide the help needed by the virus-specific CTLs. When this happens, the number of CTLs also begins to decline, and the viral load increases -- because there are too few CTLs left to cope with newly-infected cells.

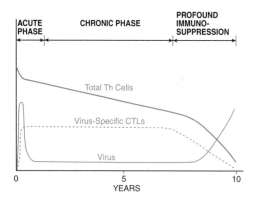

The end result is that the immune defenses are over-whelmed, and the resulting profound state of immuno-suppression leaves the patient open to unchecked infections by pathogens that would normally not be the slightest problem in a person with an intact immune system. Sadly, these "opportunistic" infections can be lethal to an AIDS patient whose immune system has been destroyed.

Why is HIV-1 able to defeat an immune system that is so successful at protecting us from most other pathogens? There are two parts to this answer. The first has to do with the nature of the virus itself. All viruses are basically pieces of genetic information (either DNA or RNA) with a protective coat. In the AIDS virus, this genetic information is in the form of RNA which, after the virus enters its target cell, is copied by an enzyme called reverse transcriptase to make a piece of "copy" DNA (cDNA). Next, the DNA of the cell is cut by an enzyme carried by the virus, and the viral cDNA is inserted (integrated) into the gap in the cellular DNA. Now comes the nasty part. Once the viral DNA has been integrated into the cellular DNA, it can just sit there. In this "latent" state, the infected cell cannot be detected by CTLs. Sometime later, in response to sig-nals that are not fully understood, the latent virus can "reactivate" to produce more viruses which can then infect other cells.

The ability to establish a latent infection that cannot be detected by CTLs is one property of HIV-1 that makes it such a problem. But it gets worse. The reverse transcriptase enzyme used to copy the viral RNA is very error-prone. It makes about one error (mutation) each time it copies a piece of viral RNA. What this means is that the new viruses that are produced by an infected cell usually are different from the virus that originally infected that cell. These mutations can have three results. First, the mutations may not change the viral structure or function at all. Second, the mutations may actually kill the virus, because they disturb some essential function (e.g., the mutation might change the reverse transcriptase so that it doesn't work). Finally (and this is the scary part), the mutations may help the virus adapt to its environment, so that it can become even more damaging.

Because of its error-prone reverse transcriptase, the virus can mutate so that a viral peptide that formerly was recognized by a CTL no longer can be recognized, or no longer can be presented by the MHC molecule that the CTL had been restricted to recognize. When such mutations occur, that CTL will be useless against cells infected with the mutant virus, and new CTLs that recognize another viral peptide will have to be activated. Meanwhile, the virus that has escaped from surveillance by the obsolete CTL is replicating like crazy, and every time it infects a new cell, it mutates again. The bottom line is that the mutation rate of the AIDS virus is so high that it can effectively stay one step ahead of CTLs or antibodies directed against it.

So the properties of HIV-1 that make it so deadly are its ability to establish an undetectable, latent infection, and its high mutation rate. But that's only half the story. The other part has to do with the cells HIV-1 infects. This virus specifically targets cells of the immune system: helper T cells, macrophages, and dendritic cells. The "docking" protein that HIV-1 binds to when it infects a cell is our old friend CD4, the co-receptor protein found in large numbers on the surfaces of helper T cells. This protein is also expressed on macrophages and dendritic cells, although they have fewer CD4 molecules on their surfaces. This is really insidious, because when HIV-1 infects these immune system cells, it either disrupts their function, kills the cells, or makes them targets for killing by CTLs that recognize them as being virus-infected. So the very cells that are needed by the adaptive immune system to activate CTLs and to provide them with help are damaged or destroyed by the virus. This killing (either directly or indirectly) of helper T cells and APCs leads to the immunosuppression that eventually results in the death of the patient.

In summary, the symptoms of an HIV-1 infection are the result of the virus's ability to slowly destroy the immune system of the patient, leading to a state of profound immunosuppression. The virus is able to do this because it can establish a latent, "stealth" infection, because it has a high mutation rate, and because it preferentially infects and disables the very immune system cells that would normally defend against it.

CANCER AND THE IMMUNE SYSTEM

In this, our last lecture, we are going to talk about the interactions that take place between cancer cells and the immune system. I suspect that some of you have not yet had a cancer course, so I think I'd better start by talking a bit about cancer cells. After all, it's important to know the enemy.

PROTO-ONCOGENES AND ANTI-ONCOGENES

It is thought that most cancers arise when a single cell suffers mutations in normal cellular genes. These genes are generally lumped into two categories: genes that promote the growth and spread (metastasis) of cancer cells (the proto-oncogenes), and genes that normally protect against cancer-causing mutations (the anti-oncogenes). When expressed appropriately, unmutated proto-oncogenes perform important functions in a normal cell. For example, they may be turned on early in development of the fetus to promote rapid cell proliferation. Because an adult human is made up of about ten trillion cells, a lot of proliferation must take place between the time we are a fertilized egg and the time we are full grown. So appropriate cell proliferation is a good thing.

On the other hand, if proto-oncogenes are turned on inappropriately (e.g., at too high a level or at the wrong time), cells that should not proliferate can be induced to do so, and cancer can result. To protect against mutations that inappropriately activate proto-oncogenes, Mother Nature has equipped cells with anti-oncogenes whose products can sense that the cell has gone "out of control" and can take appropriate measures (e.g., trigger the cell to die by apoptosis). Where things get dangerous is when proto-oncogenes are mutated, so that the cell can take on the characteristics of a cancer cell, and anti-oncogenes are mutated so

that the cell can't defend itself against these activated proto-oncogenes. In fact, the reason that cancer is generally a disease of the old is that it usually takes a long time to accumulate the multiple mutations required to enable the proto-oncogenes and disable the anti-oncogenes.

One of the hallmarks of a cancer cell is a genetically unstable condition in which genes are constantly mutating. As a result of this rapid genetic variation, most tumors consist of a mixture of cells with different mutations. This high mutation rate allows cancer cells to "evolve," so that they can acquire the characteristics of full-blown, metastatic cancer cells, and can evade the body's defense mechanisms. One gene that is designed to keep this from happening is called p53. This anti-oncogene has been termed the "guardian of the genome," because its job is to sense when mutations have occurred in cellular genes. If these mutations are not extensive, p53 stops the cell from proliferating until the mutations can be repaired. However, if there is severe genetic damage, p53 triggers apoptosis, and the errant cell is eliminated. One indication of the importance of p53 is that this anti-oncogene is inactivated (because of mutations) in a large proportion of human tumors. Interestingly, scientists have now created mice with mutant p53 genes. In contrast to normal mice which rarely get cancer, mice that lack p53 usually die of cancer before they are seven months old. So, if you are ever asked to give up one gene, don't pick p53!

STAGES IN THE LIFE OF A CANCER CELL

Let's take a look at the changes that occur as a normal cell accumulates mutations and becomes a cancer cell. As you will see, there are many obstacles that a "wannabe" cancer cell must overcome. First, it must escape from growth control mechanisms that normally keep cell proliferation in check. Most cells in an adult human are not growing. For example, when the cells in your kidney have proliferated to make that organ the right size, these cells receive negative, "don't proliferate," signals from surrounding cells and tissues, and they stop proliferating. Unfortunately, as time goes by, a kidney cell may undergo mutations that disrupt the signaling pathways which convey the "don't grow" signal, and the cell may begin to proliferate. Usually this unnatural growth will be sensed by anti-oncogenes like p53 within the cell, and the cell will be instructed to die by apoptosis. This type of internal surveillance is probably sufficient to deal with most of the wannabes.

Occasionally, however, due to mutations in oncogenes and anti-oncogenes, human cells begin to proliferate inappropriately. If you look carefully at your face, for example, you may see the result of inappropriate proliferation -- what doctors call "benign growths." The older you get, the more of these you will notice, because they result from mutations that accumulate over time. An old guy like me has lots of them! What keeps these cells from making a huge growth on your face is that they haven't figured out how to overcome the next obstacle for wannabe cancer cells -- the lack of a sufficient blood supply. You see, cells get their nourishment and growth factors from the blood, and as a result, no living cell in your body is more than about two millimeters from a blood vessel. So for a wannabe cancer cell to proliferate into a mass that is larger than about two millimeters, it must be able to secrete molecules (angiogenic factors) that recruit new blood vessels into the growing mass. Most wannabe cells can't do this, so most growths remain quite small. However, every once in a while, a wannabe cell may suffer additional mutations that result in the secretion of angiogenic factors and the recruitment of new blood vessels. When this happens, the growth can get quite large.

I think we all have an old uncle who has a big growth like this on his face. Fortunately, such a growth is usually still benign, and if it gets too big or obnoxious, a dermatologist can remove it. The growth is considered benign because it's growing very slowly, and because the wannabe cells have not learned the deadliest of their tricks -- how to metastasize. To metastasize, cells must suffer further mutations that allow them to secrete enzymes which can break down the membranes and structures that separate the growth from the blood stream. If these mutations occur, the wannabe cells can leave the original site and travel (metastasize) to other parts of the body. At this point the cells are dangerous, because although a skilled surgeon can often remove a primary tumor, cancers that have metastasized are frequently fatal.

CLASSIFICATION OF CANCER CELLS

Cancer cells can be grouped into two general categories: non-blood-cell cancers (usually referred to as "solid tumors") and blood-cell cancers. Solid tumors are further classified according to the cell type from which they arise. Carcinomas, the most common tumors in humans, are cancers of epithelial cells, and include lung, breast, colon, and cervical cancer, among others. These cancers generally kill by metastasizing to vital organs, where they grow and crowd the organ until it can no longer function properly. Humans also get cancers of the connective and structural tissues, although these "sarcomas" are relatively rare compared to carcinomas. Perhaps the best known example of a sarcoma is bone cancer (osteosarcoma). You may remember that one of the Kennedy boys had this type of malignancy.

Blood-cell cancers make up the other class of human cancers, and the most frequent of these are leukemias and lymphomas. Blood-cell cancers arise when descendants of blood stem cells, which normally should mature into lymphocytes or myeloid cells (e.g., neutrophils) stop maturing, and just continue proliferating. In a real sense, these blood cells refuse to "grow up" -- and that's the problem. In leukemia, the immature cells fill up the bone marrow and prevent other blood cells from maturing. As a result, the patient usually dies from anemia (due to a scarcity of red blood cells) or from infections (due to a scarcity of immune system cells). In lymphoma, the immature cells form solid tumors in lymph nodes, which can then metastasize to vital organs. Lymphoma patients usually succumb to infections or organ malfunction.

Lymphoma or leukemia is sometimes the result of a mistake in the VDJ recombinase activity that normally is used to create antibody and T cell receptor diversity. When mistakes are made, a proto-oncogene can recombine with a gene that has a strong promoter (frequently an antibody gene), with the result that the proto-oncogene is turned on inappropriately. Some of these proto-oncogenes function as "master genes" that can influence the expression of many other cellular genes. In a single stroke, they can activate other proto-oncogenes and inactivate anti-oncogenes. This type of mutation frequently results in <u>acute</u> lymphoma or leukemia -- diseases that can kill quickly, usually within months. Other mistakes in recombination activate proto-oncogenes that cause cells either to proliferate or to refuse to die by apoptosis. This type of mutation can extend the normal life span of the cell, and increase the probability that enough additional mutations will accumulate to turn the cell into a full-blown cancer cell. Recombination mistakes of this type frequently lead to <u>chronic</u> leukemia or lymphoma -- diseases that can take years to run their course.

There is another way to classify human cancers: spontaneous and virus-associated. This classification is especially useful in evaluating the importance of immune surveillance against cancer, because as you will see, immune surveillance is very different in these two cases. Most human tumors are called spontaneous, because they arise when a single cell accumulates a collection of mutations that causes it to acquire the properties of a metastatic cancer cell. These mutations can result from errors that are made when cellular DNA is copied to be passed down to daughters cells, or from the effect of mutagenic compounds (called carcinogens) that are byproducts of normal cellular metabolism or that are present in the air we breathe and the food we eat. Mutations can also be caused by radiation (including UV light) or by errors in recombination. As we go through life, these mutations occur "spontaneously," but there are certain factors that can <u>accelerate</u> the rate of mutation: cigarette smoking, a fatty diet, an increased radiation exposure from living at high altitude, working in a plutonium processing plant, etc.

Virus-associated cancer is also "spontaneous" in the sense that mutations caused by errors in DNA copying, carcinogens, and radiation may also be involved. What sets virus-associated cancers apart is that they have, as an additional accelerating factor, a viral infection. For example, most human cervical cancers have, as an accelerating factor, infection by the human papilloma virus. This sexually-transmitted virus infects cells that line the uterine cervix, and expresses in these cells viral proteins that can functionally inactivate anti-oncogenes such as p53. Likewise, hepatitis B virus can establish a chronic infection of liver cells, can inactivate p53, and can act as an accelerating factor for liver cancer. Epstein Barr virus (which

also causes infectious mononucleosis) can immortalize B cells and cause them to proliferate. This increases the probability that errors will be made in VDJ recombination, leading to malignancies like Burkitt's lymphoma.

The hallmark of virus-associated cancer is that only a small fraction of infected individuals will get cancer, yet for those who do, virus or viral genes can usually be recovered from their tumors. For example, only a small percentage of women infected with human papilloma virus ever get cancer of the cervix, yet human papilloma virus DNA can be recovered from over 90% of all cervical carcinomas. The reason for this, of course, is that the virus can't cause cancer by itself -- it can only accelerate the process that involves the accumulation of cancer-causing mutations.

IMMUNE SURVEILLANCE AGAINST CANCER

From this introduction, it should be clear that powerful defenses exist <u>within the cell</u> to deal harshly with most wannabe cancer cells. Whether or not the immune system also plays a major role in protecting us against the majority of human cancers is not nearly so clear. There are, of course, many anecdotal (uncontrolled) reports of a connection between the "health" of the immune system and cancer. For example, we have all heard accounts of people who have come down with cancer at times when they were under great stress, and we suppose that stress somehow reduced the strength of their immune systems and allowed a cancer cell to escape immune surveillance. We have also heard stories of patients with "incurable" cancer whose cancers vanished when they changed their diet or began to watch lots of cartoons. We imagine that their new diet or happy thoughts somehow strengthened their immune system, so that it was able to fight off the tumor.

Indeed, there is a documented connection between the "psyche" and the immune system, and also some experimental evidence which suggests that stress can weaken immune defenses against cancer. For example, my friend, Jim Cook, studies the ability of natural killer cells to kill tumor cells. For many of his studies, he uses NK cells that have been "donated" by mice. Jim tells me, however, that when he orders mice to be shipped to him from across the country, he has to let the animals recover for several weeks before he can use their cells. Newly arrived mice are so stressed by the trip that their NK cells are not very effective at killing tumor cells.

There is also good evidence that there is an increase in the incidence of cancer in humans who are immunosuppressed, either by chemotherapy or by diseases such as AIDS. Indeed, the increased incidence of lymphomas, leukemias, and virus-associated cancer in immunosuppressed humans is well documented. However, during immunosuppression, a similar increase is <u>not</u> seen in the most common of all human tumors: spontaneous tumors that are not of blood-cell origin. The same phenomenon is observed with nude mice, which are immunodeficient because they lack functional T cells. These mice have an increased incidence of lymphomas and leukemias, but do not get more spontaneous, non-blood cell cancers than normal mice. While it is possible that important immune surveillance mechanisms actually are not suppressed in these "immunosuppressed" humans and mice, these results do suggest that although immune surveillance may be involved in defending against virus-associated and blood-cell cancers, it probably is not a significant defense against most human tumors.

To try to understand why immune surveillance might be more effective against certain types of cancer than against others, let's examine the roles that various immune system cells may play in surveillance against cancer, keeping in mind that different kinds of cancer may be viewed very differently by these cells.

IMMUNE SURVEILLANCE BY MACROPHAGES AND NK CELLS

Two types of cells that may provide surveillance against cancer are macrophages and natural killer cells. Many tumor cells have receptors on their surfaces for tumor necrosis factor, and when TNF binds to these receptors, it can signal tumor cells to commit suicide by apoptosis. Hyperactivated macrophages secrete TNF, and express it on their surfaces. Either form of TNF can kill certain types of tumor cells in the test tube. This brings up the interesting point that what happens in the test tube is not always the same as what happens in the animal. For example, there are mouse sarcomas that are very resistant to killing by TNF in the test tube. In contrast, when mice that have these same sarcomas are treated with TNF, the tumors are rapidly killed. Studies

of this phenomenon showed that the reason TNF is able to kill the tumor when it is in the animal is that TNF actually attacks the blood vessels that feed the tumor, cutting off the blood supply, and causing the tumor cells to starve to death. This type of death is called "necrosis" and it was this observation that led scientists to name this cytokine "tumor necrosis factor."

There are also examples of cancer therapies in humans in which activated macrophages are likely to play a major role in tumor rejection. One such therapy involves injecting the tumor with BCG, a weakened form of the bacterium that causes tuberculosis. BCG hyperactivates macrophages, and when it is injected directly into a tumor (e.g., a melanoma), the tumor fills up with highly activated macrophages that can destroy the cancer. In fact, one of the standard treatments for bladder cancer is injections of BCG -- a treatment which is quite effective in eliminating superficial tumors, probably through the action of hyperactivated macrophages.

How do macrophages tell the difference between normal and cancer cells? The answer is not known, but the suspicion is that macrophages recognize tumor cells that have unusual cell surface molecules. One of the duties of macrophages in the spleen is to test red blood cells to see if they have become damaged or old. Macrophages use their sense of "feel" to tell which red cells are past their prime, and when they find an old one, they eat it. What macrophages feel for is a fat molecule called phosphotidyl-serine. This particular fat is usually found on the inside of young red cells, but flips to the outside when the cells get old. Like old red blood cells, tumor cells also tend to have unusual surface molecules, and in fact, some express phosphotidyl-serine on their surfaces. It is believed that the abnormal expression of surface molecules on tumor cells allows activated macrophages to differentiate between cancer cells and normal cells.

Natural killer cells also can kill some tumor cells in the test tube. They do this in the same two ways that CTLs kill virus-infected cells. First, NK cells can use perforin to poke a hole in the tumor cell membrane, and can secrete enzymes that trigger apoptosis. In addition, NK cells can express Fas ligand on their surfaces, and when this protein binds the Fas protein on tumor cells, apoptosis of the tumor cell can be triggered. Like macrophages, NK cells seem to select their tumor targets on the basis of unusual surface molecules. In addition to being able to kill tumor cells in the test tube, there is also evidence that NK cells can kill cancer cells in the body. However, these experiments are difficult to interpret, because it is not clear whether NK cells actually do the killing, or whether they simply cooperate by providing cytokines to other cells that kill (e.g., macrophages).

Now there are a number of advantages to having macrophages and NK cells provide surveillance against wannabe cancer cells that look funny on the outside. First, unlike CTLs that would take a week or more to get cranked up, macrophages and NK cells are quick-acting. This is an important consideration, because the more time that abnormal cells have to proliferate, the higher is the likelihood that they will mutate to take on the characteristics of metastatic cancer cells. In addition, once a tumor is large, it is much more difficult for killer cells to deal with. So you would like the weapons that protect against wannabe cancer cells to be ready to go as soon as the cells start to get a little weird.

Second, you would like for the weapons to be focused on diverse targets, because a single target (e.g., the MHC-peptide combination seen by a T cell) can mutate and therefore become invisible. Both NK cells and macrophages recognize diverse target structures, so the chances of them being fooled by a single mutation is small. Moreover, NK cells and macrophages are located out in the tissues where most tumors arise, so they can intercept cancer cells at an early stage. With immune surveillance, as with real estate, location is everything.

NK cells also have the advantage that they don't need to be activated to kill -- the recognition of the correct target structure on a cancer cell seems to be enough. In contrast, macrophages need to be hyperactivated before they can kill cancer cells, so if a wannabe cancer cell arises at a site of inflammation where macrophages are already hyperactivated, that's great. But if there's no inflammatory reaction going on, macrophages will probably remain in a resting state and simply ignore cancer cells. Fortunately, NK cells produce cytokines like IFN-γ that are involved in activating macrophages. In fact, one of the major functions of NK cells is to provide cytokines to other immune system cells. So if NK cells become irritated due to the presence of cancer cells, they can secrete cytokines that help hyperactivate macrophages, and these hyperactivated macrophages can then secrete cytokines (e.g., TNF) that can help hyperactivate NK cells. This is a good example of the power of "networking" in the immune system.

CTLS AND VIRUS-ASSOCIATED TUMORS

Although macrophages and NK cells may provide surveillance against some cancers, the cell that has received the most attention as a weapon against cancer cells is the cytotoxic lymphocyte. Let's begin by evaluating the ability of CTLs to provide surveillance against virus-associated tumors. This will also give us a good chance to review some of the concepts you learned in earlier lectures.

Let's imagine that a woman is infected with the sexually-transmitted, human papilloma virus that can act as an accelerating agent in cervical cancer, and let's assume this is her first exposure to the virus. Upon infection, the virus will begin to replicate in the epithelial cells that line the cervix, and after a couple of days, newly-made virus will burst out of the infected cells, leaving dead cells behind. These viruses will then infect other cells of the cervix, and the cycle will continue. Meanwhile, NK cells in the area will recognize some of the virus-infected cells and kill them, and macrophages, activated by cytokines secreted by NK cells, will phagocytose some of the virus (especially virus opsonized by complement), and will help with the killing of virus-infected cells. Together, complement, NK cells, and macrophages will generate an inflammatory reaction at the site of infection, and neutrophils will be recruited from the blood to feast on the opsonized virus.

While this is going on, some virus will be carried by the lymph to nearby lymph nodes where it can infect antigen presenting cells. In these infected APCs, viral proteins will be produced, chewed up, and displayed by class I MHC molecules. Also in lymph nodes, virus will be endocytosed (a fancy form of phagocytosis) by APCs, fragmented, and displayed by class II MHC molecules. Out in the cervix, dendritic cells that have either phagocytosed free virus or have been infected by virus will, when stimulated by the inflammatory reaction in the cervix, travel to nearby lymph nodes to display viral antigens.

Helper T cells, on their normal traffic pattern through blood, lymph, and secondary lymphoid organs, will enter lymph nodes that drain the cervix via high endothelial venules. There, if they recognize viral peptides presented by class II MHC molecules on antigen presenting cells, they will be activated. Likewise, CTLs that are circulating through lymph nodes may recognize viral antigens displayed by class I MHC molecules on APCs, receive help from activated helper T cells, and become activated. Once activated, Th cells and CTLs will leave the lymph nodes via the lymph, and will recirculate. Some recirculating T cells will re-enter lymph nodes and other secondary lymphoid organs, while others will exit the blood in the area of the cervix to join in the battle that the innate immune system is waging against the viral infection. In the cervix, APCs that have been infected with or have phagocytosed virus can present viral antigens to experienced CTLs and Th cells to re-stimulate them. Re-stimulated Th cells can provide cytokines needed by the soldiers of the innate and adaptive immune systems, and re-stimulated CTLs can kill virus-infected cells in the cervix.

At the same time that CTLs are being activated, B cells will also be springing into action. Virus or fragments of virus that have been opsonized by complement will be swept into the lymph nodes that drain the cervix, and will be captured there on the surfaces of follicular dendritic cells. Virgin B cells that enter these nodes via high endothelial venules may recognize their cognate antigens, receive co-stimulation from activated helper T cells, and become activated. Once activated, most B cells will re-enter the circulation so that activated B cells will be spread around to more lymph nodes. Some B cells will travel to the spleen or bone marrow, and will produce IgM antibodies that can opsonize or neutralize the virus. Other activated B cells will migrate to lymphoid follicles where, under the influence of cytokines from activated Th cells, they can undergo somatic hypermutation to "fine tune" their receptors to more efficiently bind to viral antigens, and can class switch to produce antibody classes (e.g., IgG and IgA) that are especially appropriate for defending against viruses.

What I have just described is known as the "acute" phase of a viral infection. For many viruses (e.g., smallpox), the end result of this immune reaction is total eradication of virus from the body. After the virus has been vanquished, the inflammatory reaction dies down, neutrophils die off, and those macrophages that have not died in battle go back to their resting state. Deprived of antigen to re-stimulate them or exhausted by exertion, most B and T cells die, but some remain as memory cells to protect against future attacks by the same virus.

With human papilloma virus, however, the battle frequently has a different outcome, because this particular virus can establish a "latent" infection in some of the cells of the cervix. How latent infections are maintained is still quite a mystery, but latently-infected cells are the ones that can go on to become cancer cells, and all viruses that are cancer-associated are able to establish latent infections. Although cells that are latently infected with human papilloma virus continue to produce several viral proteins, for some reason these cells are invisible to the immune system. In the laboratory, expression of MHC class I molecules and the TAP transporter is downregulated in cells infected with human papilloma virus, and it is presumed that this may also happen in latently infected cells in the body, helping them to hide from immune surveillance. In any case, the net result is that although the acute phase of the viral infection efficiently activates CTLs, and although CTLs that recognize viral antigens are present as memory cells, nevertheless they are unable to kill these latently infected cells. Of course, if latently infected cells "reactivate" (as they may do from time to time) and begin to produce more viruses that infect more cells, memory CTLs can be reactivated to keep this infection under control. In fact, you might argue that without CTLs, more cells would have a chance to become latently infected, and this may be one reason why immunosuppressed humans have a higher than normal rate of virus-associated tumors.

The bottom line, however, is that although CTLs are great against an acute viral infection, once the virus has established a latent state, CTLs can only wait for the virus to reactivate. As a result, latently infected cells that may eventually become cancerous usually go undetected by CTLs.

CTLS AND SPONTANEOUS TUMORS

Next let's evaluate the role that CTLs may play in surveillance against tumors that are not virus-associated. Let's imagine that a heavy smoker finally accumulates enough mutations in the cells of his lungs to turn one of them into a metastatic tumor cell. Remember, it only takes one bad cell to make a cancer. And let's imagine that because of these mutations, this cell expresses proteins that could be recognized as foreign by Th cells and CTLs. Proteins with this property are usually referred to as "tumor antigens." Now let me ask you a question: Where were the naive T cells while this tumor was growing in the lung? That's right. They were circulating through the blood, lymph, and secondary lymphoid organs. Do they leave this circulation pattern to enter the tissues of the lung? No, not until after they have been activated.

So right away we have a traffic problem. To make self tolerance work, Mother Nature set up the traffic system so that naive T cells don't get out into the tissues where they might encounter self antigens that were not present in the thymus during tolerance induction. As a result, it's hard to imagine how virgin T cells would ever "see" tumor antigens expressed in the lung -- because they just don't go there. What we have here is a serious conflict between the need to preserve tolerance of self (and avoid autoimmune disease) and the need to provide surveillance against tumors that arise, as most tumors do, in the tissues. And tolerance wins.

Now, sometimes virgin T cells do disobey the traffic laws and wander out into the tissues. So you might imagine that this kind of adventure could give T cells a chance to look at the tumor that's growing on this guy's lung, and be activated. But wait! What is required for T cell activation? T cells must see their cognate antigen presented by MHC molecules and they must receive co-stimulatory signals. Since CTLs recognize antigens that are produced within a cell and presented by class I MHC, the tumor cell itself must present the tumor antigens. But is that lung tumor cell going to be able to provide the co-stimulation required for activation? I don't think so! This isn't an antigen presenting cell, after all. It's a plain old lung cell, and lung cells usually don't express co-stimulatory molecules like B7. Consequently, if a renegade, virgin CTL breaks the traffic laws, enters the lung, and recognizes a tumor antigen, that CTL will most likely be anergized or killed -- because the tumor cell cannot provide the co-stimulation the CTL needs. Again we see a conflict between tolerance induction and tumor surveillance. This two-key system of specific recognition and co-stimulation was set up so that T cells which recognize self antigens out in the tissues, but which do not receive proper co-stimulation, will be anergized or killed to prevent autoimmunity. Unfortunately, this same two-key system makes it very difficult for CTLs to be activated by tumor cells.

Now, you may be thinking that Mother Nature really blew it by designing a system in which tumor surveillance is in conflict with self tolerance. But remember that the main concern in setting up this system was to protect us against disease (both microbial and autoimmune) until we are old enough to produce and rear our offspring. Because cancer is mainly a disease that afflicts older persons, surveillance against cancer was not a high priority (i.e., not of selective value) during evolution of the immune system.

So the bottom line is that a CTL would have to perform "unnatural acts" to be activated by a tumor out in the tissues: It would have to break the traffic laws, and somehow avoid being anergized or killed. This could happen, of course, but it would be very inefficient in comparison to activation of CTLs in response to a viral infection. Alternatively, tumor cells could metastasize to a lymph node, and T cells might be activated there, but by the time this happens, the game is probably over.

The inefficient activation of CTLs by tumor cells is doubly troublesome. If CTLs eventually are activated, they will probably have a large (and perhaps metastatic) tumor to deal with. Even worse, the tumor cells will have had plenty of time to mutate to evade detection by CTLs. Cancer cells mutate like crazy, and there are many different mutations that can prevent recognition or presentation of tumor antigens. For example, the gene encoding the tumor antigen itself can mutate so that the tumor antigen is no longer recognized by the CTL or no longer fits properly into the groove of the MHC molecule for presentation. In addition, tumor cells can mutate so that they do not produce the MHC molecule that CTLs are restricted to recognize. This happens quite frequently -- about 15% of the tumors that have been examined have turned off expression of at least one of their MHC molecules. Further, in the tumor cell, genes that encode the LMP proteins or the TAP transporters can mutate, so that tumor antigens will not be efficiently processed or transported for loading onto class I MHC molecules. This high mutation rate is the tumor's greatest advantage over the immune system, and it usually can keep tumor cells one step ahead of surveillance by CTLs. Thus, when it occurs, CTL surveillance is probably a case of "too little, too late."

Okay, so CTLs probably don't provide serious surveillance against non-blood-cell, spontaneous tumors. That's a real bummer, because these make up the majority of human tumors. But what about blood-cell cancers like leukemia and lymphoma? Maybe CTLs are useful against them. After all, immunosuppressed humans and mice do have higher frequencies of leukemia and lymphoma than do normal humans and mice. This suggests that there might be something fundamentally different about the way the immune system views tumors in tissues and organs versus the way it views blood cells that have become cancer cells. What might these differences be? Let's take a look.

One of the difficulties that CTLs have in providing surveillance against tumors that arise in tissues is that these tumors simply are not on the normal traffic pattern of virgin T cells, and it's hard to imagine how a CTL could be activated by an antigen it doesn't see. In contrast, most blood-cell cancers are found in the blood, lymph, and secondary lymphoid organs, and this is ideal for viewing by CTLs, which are passing through these areas all the time. Thus, in the case of blood-cell cancers, the traffic patterns of cancer cells and virgin T cells actually intersect. Moreover, in contrast to tumors in tissues, which usually are unable to supply the co-stimulation required for activation of virgin T cells, some cancerous blood cells actually express high levels of B7, and therefore can provide the necessary co-stimulation. These properties of blood-cell cancers suggest that CTLs might provide surveillance against some of them. Unfortunately, this surveillance must be incomplete, because people still get leukemias and lymphomas.

My conclusion is that CTLs, by their nature, are not very good at providing surveillance against cancer cells. Nevertheless, immunologists have shown that CTLs from some cancer patients can kill tumor cells in the test tube. Based on these findings, immunologists hope that CTLs or tumor cells can be manipulated so that CTLs will learn to kill tumor cells efficiently in the patient. Early evidence suggests that in a few cases, this may be possible. The realistic goal of this approach is to treat the "minimum residual disease" that remains after the surgeon has removed the primary tumor -- and we can all hope that these experiments will be successful. But in the mean time, eat right, be careful what you take into your lungs, and get plenty of rest.

ADCC - Antibody-dependent cellular cytotoxicity. Antibodies bind to the target, and Fc receptors on the surfaces of cytotoxic cells (e.g., macrophages and NK cells) bind to the antibodies to form a "bridge" between the target and the cytotoxic cell: antibody-directed killing.

Allergen - An antigen that causes allergies.

Anergy - A state of non-functionality.

Antigen - A rather loosely used term for the target (e.g., a viral protein) of an antibody or a T cell. To be more precise, an antibody binds to a <u>region</u> of an antigen called the epitope, and the T cell receptor binds to a peptide that is a <u>frag-ment</u> of the antigen.

APC - Antigen presenting cell -- cells like macrophages, dendritic cells, and activated B cells that can present antigen efficiently to T cells via MHC molecules, and which can supply the co-stimulatory molecules required to activate T cells.

Apoptosis - Sometimes called programmed cell death. The process by which cells commit suicide in response to prob-lems within the cell or to signals from outside the cell.

Autocrine - A fancy word for "self" (e.g., autocrine stimulation is self stimulation).

BCR - B cell receptor.

β2-microglobulin - The non-polymorphic chain of the class I MHC molecule.

Central tolerance induction - Process by which T cells with receptors that recognize abundant self antigens in the thy-mus are anergized or deleted.

Clonal selection principle - When receptors on B or T cells recognize their cognate antigen, these cells are triggered (selected) to proliferate. As a result, a clone of B or T cells with identical antigen specificities is produced.

Cognate antigen - The antigen (e.g., a bacterial protein) that a T or B cell receptor can recognize and bind to.

Co-receptor - The CD4 or CD8 molecule on T cells, or the complement receptor on B cells.

Co-stimulation - The second "key" that B and T cells need for activation.

Crosslink - Cluster together (e.g., an antigen may crosslink B cell receptors).

Cross reacts - Recognizes several different epitopes. For example, a B cell's receptors may bind to (cross react with) several different epitopes that are present on several different antigens.

CTL - Cytotoxic lymphocyte -- sometimes called a killer T cell.

Cytokines - Hormone-like messenger molecules that cells use to communicate.

Cytokine profile - The mixture of different cytokines that a cell secretes.

Cytoplasm - The liquid portion of a cell in which the organelles and the nucleus "float."

DC - Dendritic cell. This starfish-shaped cell functions as an antigen presenting cell for T cells.

DTH - Delayed type hypersensitivity. An inflammatory reaction in which Th cells recognize a specific invader, and secrete cytokines that activate and recruit innate system cells to do the killing.

Endocytosis - Similar to phagocytosis except that it begins when the thing being "eaten" binds to a receptor on the surface of the phagocytic cell: receptor-initiated phagocytosis.

Endogenous - From inside the cell.

Endoplasmic reticulum - A large sack-like structure inside the cell from which most proteins destined for transport to the cell surface begin their journey.

Endothelial cells - Cells shaped like shingles that line the insides of our blood vessels.

Epithelial cells - Cells shaped like cubes that usually form part of the barrier that separates our bodies from the out-side world.

Epitope - The region of an antigen that is recognized by B or T cell receptors.

Exogenous - From outside the cell.

Germinal center - An area in a secondary lymphoid organ in which B cells are proliferating, and are undergoing somatic hypermutation and class switching. Also known as a "<u>secondary</u> lymphoid follicle."

Hc - Heavy chain of the antibody molecule.

High endothelial venule (HEV) - A region in a blood vessel where there are high endothelial cells which allow lym-phocytes to exit the blood.

IFN-γ - Interferon gamma -- a cytokine secreted mainly by Th1 helper T cells and NK cells.

Inflammatory response - A rather general term that describes the battle that macrophages, neutrophils, and other immune system cells wage against an invader.

Interleukin - A protein (cytokine) that is used for communication between leukocytes (e.g., IL-2).

Isotype - A synonym for "class." The isotype of an antibody (e.g., IgA or IgG) is determined by the constant region of its heavy chain.

Lc - Light chain of the antibody molecule.

Leukocytes - All blood cells, white and red.

Ligand - A molecule that binds to a receptor (e.g., the Fas ligand binds to the Fas receptor protein on the surface of a cell).

Ligate - Bind to. When a receptor has bound its ligand, it is said to be "ligated."

Lymph - The liquid that "leaks" out of blood vessels into the tissues.

Lymphocytes - T cells and B cells.

Lymphoid follicle - A region of a secondary lymphoid organ that contains follicular dendritic cells embedded in a sea of B cells.

M cell - A cell that crowns a Peyer's patch, and which specializes in sampling antigen from the intestine.

MALT - Mucosal associated lymphoid tissues. Secondary lymphoid organs that are associated with mucosa (e.g., Peyers patches and tonsils).

MHC proteins - Proteins encoded by the major histocompatibility complex (the region of a chromosome that includes a "complex" of genes involved in antigen presentation).

MHC restriction - Survival in the thymus is "restricted" to T cells whose receptors recognize antigen presented by MHC molecules.

Microbe - A generic term that includes bacteria and viruses.

Mucosa - The tissues and associated mucus that protect exposed surfaces such as the gastrointestinal and respiratory tracts.

Necrosis - Cell death, typically caused by burns or other trauma. This type of cell death (as opposed to apoptotic cell death) usually results in the contents of the cell being dumped into the tissues where it can cause damage.

Negative selection - Synonym for "central tolerance induction."

Opsonize - "Decorate" with fragments of complement proteins or with antibodies.

Pathogen - A disease-causing agent (e.g., a bacterium or a virus).

Peptides - Small protein fragments.

Peripheral tolerance - The mechanisms that induce self tolerance outside the thymus.

Phagocytes - Cells like macrophages and neutrophils that engulf (phagocytose) invaders.

Positive selection - Synonym for "MHC restriction."

Primary lymphoid organs - The thymus and the bone marrow.

Proliferate - Increase in number. A cell proliferates by dividing into two daughter cells, which then can divide again to give four cells, and so on.

Proteasome - A multi-protein complex in the cell that chops proteins up into small pieces.

Secondary lymphoid organs - Organs like the lymph nodes, Peyer's patches, and the spleen where activation of naive B and T cells takes place.

Secrete - Export out of the cell.

TCR - T cell receptor.

Th - Helper T cell.

TNF - Tumor necrosis factor -- a cytokine secreted mainly by macrophages and helper T cells.

Virgin (naive) lymphocytes - B and T cells which have never been activated.